Advances and Technical Standards in Neurosurgery

Volume 39

Editor-in-Chief

J. Schramm, Bonn

Series Editors

N. Akalan, Ankara
V. Benes Jr., Prague
C. di Rocco, Roma
V.V. Dolenc, Ljubljana
J. Lobo Antunes, Lisbon
J.D. Pickard, Cambridge
Z.H. Rappaport, Petah Tiqva
M. Sindou, Lyon

For further volumes
http://www.springer.com/series/578

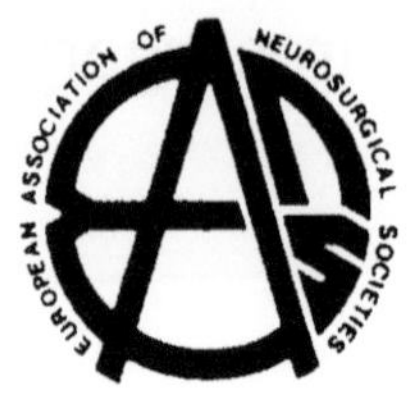

Sponsored by the
European Association of Neurosurgical Societies

Nejat Akalan • Concezio Di Rocco

Editors

Pediatric Epilepsy Surgery

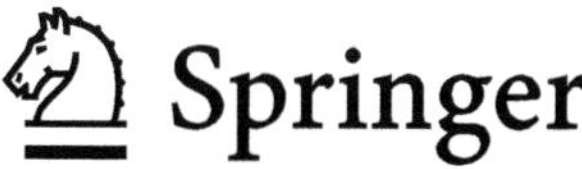 Springer

Editors
Nejat Akalan
Fac. Medicine, Dept. Neurosurgery
Hacettepe University
Sihhiye, Ankara
Turkey

Concezio Di Rocco
Ist. Neurochirurgia, Dipto. Neuroscienze
Università Cattolica del Sacro Cuore
Roma
Italy

ISBN 978-3-7091-1675-3   ISBN 978-3-7091-1360-8 (eBook)
DOI 10.1007/978-3-7091-1360-8
Springer Wien Heidelberg New York Dordrecht London

Contents

Advances

New Insight on the Mechanisms of Epileptogenesis in the Developing Brain

Hana Kubova, Katarzyna Lukasiuk, and Asla Pitkänen

Contents

H. Kubova
Department of Developmental Epileptology,
Institute of Physiology, Academy of Sciences of the Czech Republic,
Vídeňská 1083, Prague 4, CZ-142 20, Czech Republic
e-mail: kubova@biomed.cas.cz

K. Lukasiuk
Department of Molecular and Cellular Neurobiology,
The Nencki Institute of Experimental Biology, Polish Academy of Sciences,
3 Pasteur St., 02-093, Warsaw, Poland
e-mail: k.lukasiuk@nencki.gov.pl

A. Pitkänen (✉)
Department of Neurobiology,
A. I. Virtanen Institute for Molecular Sciences, University of Eastern Finland,
P. O. Box 1627, FIN-70 211, Kuopio, Finland

Department of Neurology, Kuopio University Hospital,
P. O. Box 1777, FIN-70211, Kuopio, Finland
e-mail: asla.pitkanen@uef.fi

N. Akalan, C. Di Rocco (eds.), *Pediatric Epilepsy Surgery,*
Advances and Technical Standards in Neurosurgery,
DOI 10.1007/978-3-7091-1360-8_1, © Springer-Verlag Wien 2012

Abstract The incidence of epilepsy is at its highest in childhood and seizures can persist for a lifetime. As brain tissue from pediatric patients with epilepsy is rarely available, the analysis of molecular and cellular changes during epileptogenesis, which could serve as targets for treatment approaches, has to rely largely on the analysis of tissue from animal models. However, these data have to be analyzed in the context of the developmental stage when the insult occurs. Here we review the current status of the available animal models, the molecular analysis done in these models, as well as treatment attempts to prevent epileptogenesis in the immature brain. Considering that epilepsy is one of the major childhood neurological diseases, it is remarkable how little is known on epileptogenesis in the immature brain at a molecular level. It is a true challenge for the future to expand the armamentarium of clinically relevant animal models, and systematic analysis of molecular and cellular data to enhance the probability of developing syndrome specific antiepileptogenic treatments and biomarkers for acquired pediatric epileptogenesis.

Keywords Development • Epileptogenesis • Epilepsy • Hypoxia • Ischemia • Stroke • Traumatic brain injury • Video-EEG monitoring

Introduction

Meta-analysis of the epidemiology of epilepsy revealed that the median incidence of epilepsy in childhood (0–14 years of age) is 82/100,000/year, which was significantly higher than that in the adult population (15–59 years), with an incidence rate of 34.7/100,000/year [59]. Sillanpää and colleagues estimated that the number of children and adolescents in Europe with active epilepsy is 0.9 million (prevalence 4.5–5.0/1,000) [35].

In pediatric neurology, epilepsies represent a diverse group of disorders that manifest in seizures with disparate semiology, prognosis, and pharmacological responsiveness and which are often unrelated to the type of epileptogenic brain insult [82]. According to a theory of *critical developmental periods*, the sensitivity of the immature brain to unfavorable conditions such as hypoxia, prolonged epileptiform activity (e.g., status epilepticus), or brain inflammation is highly age-dependent, and the disabling consequences in adulthood appear to be linked to the maturation stage at the time of the occurrence of an insult [95]. Moreover, the phenotypic characteristics of epilepsy, such as seizure type and sensitivity to treatments, can change with maturation. Therefore, modeling-acquired epileptogenesis in the immature brain using clinically relevant brain insults has been a major challenge.

"Epileptogenesis" and "latency period" are often used synonymously as operational terms that refer to a time period between the insult and the occurrence of the first unprovoked seizure. Evidence is accumulating to show that the neurobiological changes that occur during the latency period continue to progress, even after epilepsy diagnosis [87, 89]. Therefore, a revised definition for epileptogenesis has recently been suggested [36, 86]. The major difference from the previous definition is that epileptogenesis extends from the latency period to include the epilepsy phase. Thus, the term *"epileptogenesis"* is defined as the development and extension of tissue capable of generating spontaneous seizures, including (a) development of an epileptic condition and (b) progression after the condition is established. To describe the effect of treatments, the term *"disease or syndrome modification"* was suggested, which refers to a process that alters the development or progression of a "disease," in this case epilepsy (either epileptic disease or epilepsy syndrome). Disease- or syndrome-modifying interventions might be "antiepileptogenic," which refers to a process that counteracts the effects of epileptogenesis, including (a) prevention (lower percentage of subjects develop epilepsy), (b) seizure modification (e.g., shorter and less frequent seizures), and (c) cure. These interventions could also modify comorbidities by reducing or preventing deleterious nonepileptic functional changes in the brain (e.g., memory, emotional behavior).

A large number of studies in experimental models show that the immature rodent brain is more susceptible to induced seizures triggered with chemoconvulsants than is the adult brain. However, the susceptibility to induced seizures at a given stage of development appears to depend on the mechanisms of action of the chemoconvulsant. Also, the semiology of *induced seizures* changes with age as certain behavioral seizure types can or cannot be induced at a specific developmental stage. Also, the ED_{50} for a chemoconvulsant changes with maturation (for review, see [63, 116]).

On the other hand, for a long time the immature brain was considered resistant against acquired epileptogenesis, that is, epileptogenesis induced by brain insults. In recent years, several laboratories have provided evidence that the insults that are highly epileptogenic in the adult brain can also trigger epileptogenesis in immature animals (for review, see [101]). However, in the majority of the available animal models, the epilepsy phenotype includes only complex partial seizures with or without secondary generalization, and, thus, the diversity of various seizure types characteristic to pediatric epilepsy is only partially reproduced. As the progress in modeling age-specific epilepsies or epileptic encephalopathies has been slow, there is a good reason to ask: Where are we now? Do we currently have any relevant and reproducible models of epileptogenesis for pediatric epilepsies and, in particular, for those that are age-dependent?

The criteria for becoming a valid model for pediatric epilepsies and encephalopathies are challenging. The epileptogenic process should result in unprovoked seizures that (1) occur within a certain period of postnatal development; (2) produce an epilepsy phenotype that resembles that in humans, including a specific seizure semiology; (3) present syndrome-specific pathologic, electroencephalographic (EEG), and imaging abnormalities; (4) possess a pharmacological sensitivity corresponding to that in humans; (5) result in developmental regression or retardation; (6) have specific behavioral/cognitive sequelae; and, finally, (7) present syndrome-specific genetic mutations (see [107]). Valid animal models of epileptogenesis and epilepsy should provide a useful tool for investigating the molecular and cellular mechanisms of epileptogenesis to identify biomarkers, to test new antiepileptogenic and antiepileptic drugs, and to advance the development of new diagnostic and therapeutic strategies. Therefore, the incentives for the challenge of developing models for epileptogenesis in the developing brain are high and motivating.

Modeling Acquired Epilepsy in Immature Rodents

A summary of models is presented in Table 1.

Status Epilepticus

Status epilepticus (SE) is defined as a continuous unremitting seizure lasting longer than 30 min, or as discontinuous seizures lasting more than 30 min without a return to normal function between seizures [72]. Epidemiological data show that the incidence of convulsive SE in childhood is between 17 and 23/100,000/year [103]. Even though the data are variable, there is agreement that SE is a risk factor for epileptogenesis later (see [84]).

Chemically Induced SE

Chemically induced SE represents the most frequently used insult to trigger epileptogenesis in the immature brain. Experimental studies have now demonstrated that the consequences of SE are largely, but not exclusively, dependent on the stage of development at the time of occurrence of SE as well as on the severity and duration of SE (for review, see [70, 101]). Other factors such as genetic background, method of induction of SE, treatment during SE, or additional pathophysiological conditions such as body temperature and co-occurring inflammation also contribute to the outcome.

Pilocarpine

For a long time the immature brain was considered to be resistant to SE-induced epileptogenesis. However, data from several laboratories have now demonstrated that systemic administration of pilocarpine (with or without lithium) can produce SE in a reproducible way within the first 2 weeks of life [4, 15, 44]. The progress in modeling is a result of the development of new technologies for seizure detection, such as computerized video-EEG monitoring for small laboratory animals, which has become more available and more affordable. More accurate monitoring could overcome the problems related to video monitoring only, as also the subclinical electrographic seizures with minor behavioral manifestations could be detected. Priel and collaborators [90] used only video

Table 1 Summary of in vitro and in vivo changes in excitability in different animal models of acquired pediatric epilepsy

Model	Species, age, strain, preparation	Seizure susceptibility in vitro and/or in vivo	Epilepsy					
			Animals with epilepsy (%)	Latency to spontaneous sz	Sz frequency	Sz duration (s)	Epileptiform spiking or EDs in EEG	Reference
SE – pilocarpine or Li-pilocarpine*								
In vivo*	Rat, P7–120, Wistar (only video monitoring used for seizure detection)	n.d.	Convulsive spontaneous seizures demonstrated only in animals P18 and older	Decreased with age at SE P18–P24 36.5±24.8 days P25–P35 23.2±10.3 days	Increased with age at SE and progressed with time after SE 4 months after SE Seizure frequency 4 months after SE: P18–P24 2.5±1.3 sz P25–P35 3.6±2.0 sz	n.d.	n.d.	Priel et al. [90]
In vivo	Rat, 2, 3, 4 weeks, Wistar, (video-EEG monitoring of rats with behavioral seizures)	n.d.	Analysis ≥3 months post-SE 2 weeks (27.3 %) 3 weeks (72.7 %) 4 weeks (75.0 %)	n.d.	n.d.	n.d.	n.d.	Sankar et al. [97]

(continued)

Table 1 (continued)

Model	Species, age, strain, preparation	Seizure susceptibility in vitro and/or in vivo	Epilepsy					Reference
			Animals with epilepsy (%)	Latency to spontaneous sz	Sz frequency	Sz duration (s)	Epileptiform spiking or EDs in EEG	
In vivo	Rat, P10, Spraque-Dawley	3–4 months after SE no effects on seizure susceptibility (seizures induced with pentylenetet-razol, picrotoxin, kainate)	n.d.	n.d.	n.d.	n.d.	n.d.	Nehlig et al. [83]
In vivo	Rat, P10, P21, adults, Spraque-Dawley	n.d.	Spontaneous seizures P10 (0 %) P21 (24 %)	n.d.	n.d.	n.d.	n.d.	Dube et al. [28]
In vivo	Rat, P12 or P25, Wistar (video-EEG monitoring) monitoring	n.d.	3 months Post-SE P12 (25 %) P25 (50 %)	n.d.	n.d.	n.d.	P12 (75 %) P25 (100 %)	Kubová et al. [61]

In vivo	Rat, P12 or P25, Wistar (video-EEG monitoring)	n.d.	5 months post- SE P12 (50 %) P25 (83.3 %) 7 months post-SE P12 (87.5 %)	n.d.	5 months P12 1.4±0.6/ days P25 10.4±3.7/ days 7 months P12 8.2±4.0/ days	5 months P12 10.6±1.5 s P25 19.3±5.5 s 7 months P12 38±15.1 s	5 months P12 (66.6 %) P25 (100 %) 7 months P12 (100 %)	Kubova (not published)
In vivo	Rat, P21, Wistar (EEG monitoring only in animals with convulsive seizures)	PPI Augmentation of dentate inhibition under ketamine anesthesia	2–4 months post-SE P21 (73 %)	n.d.	n.d.	n.d.	n.d.	Sankar et al. [98]
In vivo	Rat, P12 or P25, Wistar	Electrically induced cortical after-discharges Delayed transition into limbic seizures and increased threshold for limbic after-discharges in animals with SE	n.d.	n.d.	n.d.	n.d.	n.d.	Tsenov et al. [115]

(continued)

Table 1 (continued)

Model	Species, age, strain, preparation	Seizure susceptibility in vitro and/or in vivo	Epilepsy					Reference
			Animals with epilepsy (%)	Latency to spontaneous sz	Sz frequency	Sz duration (s)	Epileptiform spiking or EDs in EEG	
SE – kainic acid								
In vivo	Rat, P5, P10, P20, P30, and P60, Spraque-Dawley, (video-monitoring only)	At P100–P130 decreased latency to flurothyl-induced seizures in P20, P30, and P60 animals with spontaneous seizures	3 months post-SE P5 (0 %) P10 (0 %) P20 (14 %) P30 (30 %) P60 (44 %)	First seizure recorded P20 4 weeks post-SE P30 7 weeks post-SE P60 1 week post-SE	P20 1.0 sz/day P30 1.2 sz/day P60 2.4 sz/day	About 40 s in all age groups	n.d.	Stafstrom et al. [106]
In vivo	Rat, P27, Wistar (intermittent observation)	Lower number of kindling stimulations needed to reach Stage 5 in adulthood	66.7 %	n.d.	n.d.	n.d.	n.d.	Holmes and Thompson [46]
In vivo	Rat, P1, P7, P14, P24, and P75	3 months post-SE Slower development of generalized kindled seizures in P1–P14 but not in older age groups	n.d.	n.d.	n.d.	n.d.	n.d.	Lynch et al. [74]

In vitro	Rat, P1, P7, P14, P24, and P75	3 months post-SE P1–P14, enhanced paired-pulse inhibition in the dentate gyrus P21 and P24 decreased paired-pulse inhibition in the dentate gyrus	n.d.	n.d.	n.d.	n.d.	n.d.	Lynch et al. [74]
Multiple episodes of chemically induced SE								
In vivo (3 periods of SE induced with pilo-carpine)	Rat, P7, P8, P9, Wistar (EEG recordings)	n.d.	At P33, P45, P63, and P93 subclinical electrographic epileptiform activity in 100 % of animals, convulsive seizures in 10 %	n.d.	n.d.	n.d.	n.d.	Santos et al. [99]
SE – electrically induced								
In vivo	Rat, P21 and P35, Wistar (EEG monitoring only in animals with convulsive seizures)	Augmentation of dentate inhibition in P35 but not in P21 animals	Spontaneous seizures at 2–4 months post-SE P21 (11 %) P35 (100 %)	n.d.	n.d.	n.d.	n.d.	Sankar et al. [98]

(continued)

Table 1 (continued)

Model	Species, age, strain, preparation	Seizure susceptibility in vitro and/or in vivo	Epilepsy					Reference
			Animals with epilepsy (%)	Latency to spontaneous sz	Sz frequency	Sz duration (s)	Epileptiform spiking or EDs in EEG	
Hyperthermia-induced seizures or SE								
In vivo	Rat, P10 or P11, Spraque-Dawley Hyperthermia (~41 °C) lasting for 24 or 64 min (intermittent video-EEG monitoring)	n.d.	Intermittent monitoring 3–6 months after insult P10 (24 min) (35 %) P11 (64 min) (45 %)	In 50 % of animals seizures present already at 3 months after insult	n.d.	Behavioral seizures lasting for 6–18 s	88.2 %	Dubé et al. [29]
In vivo	Rat, P10–P11, Spraque-Dawley Hyperthermia (~41 °C) lasting for 30 min (intermittent video-EEG monitoring)	96±5 days after insult Decreased threshold for kainate-induced seizures	At 10–11 weeks after hyperthermia no spontaneous seizures	–	–	–	–	Dube et al. [28]

In vivo	Rat, P2, Wistar Ambient temperature ~45 °C until the first seizure; multiple seizures (up to 8)	Increased susceptibility to pilocarpine-induced seizures at P60–P70	n.d.	n.d.	n.d.	n.d.	n.d.	Gulec and Noyan [38]
In vitro	Rat, P10–P11, Spraque-Dawley Hyperthermic seizures (~41 °C) for 30 min (intermittent EEG monitoring)	Enhanced excitability in hippocampal-entorhinal slices at 1 week after hyperthermia	At 10–11 weeks after hyperthermia no spontaneous seizures	–	–	–	–	Dube et al. [28]
In vivo	Rat, P10, Spraque-Dawley (20 min intermittent video monitoring at P83 and EEG monitoring at P168)	n.d.	No spontaneous seizures detected				Interictal spikes in 28.6 % of animals	Scantlebbury et al. [100]

(continued)

Table 1 (continued)

Model	Species, age, strain, preparation	Seizure susceptibility in vitro and/or in vivo	Epilepsy					
			Animals with epilepsy (%)	Latency to spontaneous sz	Sz frequency	Sz duration (s)	Epileptiform spiking or EDs in EEG	Reference
Hypoxia-ischemia – ligation of common carotid artery								
In vivo	Rat, P7, Spraque-Dawley Unilateral carotid ligation with hypoxia (video-EEG monitoring)	n.d.	Up to 12 months follow-up, spontaneous seizures in 56 % (all rats with a cerebral infarct)	n.d.	Progressively increased with time after insult (0.2 sz/day at 3 months and 1.4 sz/day at 12 months after insult)	95.3±1.4 s (Racine 5) 47±3.5 s (Racine <5)	In all rats with spontaneous seizures	Kadam et al. [53]
In vivo	Rat, P7, Spraque-Dawley Unilateral carotid ligation with hypoxia Observation of seizures (6 h/week)	n.d.	Up to 24 months (40 %)	194±43 days	0.012±0.0035 sz/h	n.d.	n.d.	Williams et al. [120]
In vivo	Rat, P12–P13, Wistar Repeated cortical stimulation	2.5 months after insult Transient decrease in threshold to convulsive seizures	2.5 months after insult (23 %)	–	–	–	–	Romjin et al. [94]

In vivo	Rat, P7, Spraque-Dawley	7 and 21 days after insult No changes in susceptibility to bicucull-ine-induced seizures	–	–	–	–	–	Cataltepe et al. [14]
Hypoxia-ischemia – endothelin-1								
In vivo	Rat, P12 or P25, Wistar Intrahippocampal injection of ET-1 Video-EEG monitoring	n.d.	3 months after insult P12 (71.4 %) P25 (91.7 %)	n.d.	P12 up to 97 sz/day P25 up to 51 sz/day	P12 9.1±1.2 s P25 6.5±0.4 s	P12 92.9 % P25 91.7 %	Mateffyova et al. [75]
Hypoxia-ischemia – prolonged hypoxia								
In vivo	Rat, P10, Long-Evans Video-EEG monitoring	n.d.	>P60 (94.4 %)	About 2 week after insult	5.8±1 sz/h in posthypoxic animals 0. 1±0.06 sz/h in normoxic controls	7.32±0.12 s	n.d.	Rakhade et al. [92]

(continued)

Table 1 (continued)

Model	Species, age, strain, preparation	Seizure susceptibility in vitro and/or in vivo	Epilepsy					Reference
			Animals with epilepsy (%)	Latency to spontaneous sz	Sz frequency	Sz duration (s)	Epileptiform spiking or EDs in EEG	
In vivo	Rat, P1 or P10, Long-Evans	4 weeks No changes in susceptibility to flurothyl-induced seizures or kindling	n.d.	n.d.	n.d.	n.d.	n.d.	Jensen et al. [51]
In vivo	Rat, P1 or P10, Long-Evans	4 weeks No changes in susceptibility to flurothyl-induced seizures or kindling						
In vitro	Rat, P10–P11, Long-Evans	Hippocampal slices, at P70–P80 increased frequency of ictal discharges (low Mg^{2+}) in hypoxic animals	n.d.	n.d.	n.d.	n.d.	n.d.	Jensen et al. [52]

Infantile spasms

In vivo	Rat, P10–P12, Wistar		Monitoring for 28.5 days after infusion	n.d.	n.d.	1–2 s	Multifocal spike and sharp-wave dis-charges in 100 % of animals	Lee et al. [67]
	Intrahippocampal or cortical infusion of tetrodotoxin		Brief behavioral spasms in 31.6 % of animals with cortical and 31.2 % of animals with hippocampal infusion					
	EEG monitoring							
In vivo	Rat, Spraque-Dawley	n.d.	At P4–P9, spasms in 100 % of animals	n.d.	n.d.	n.d.	Spikes, runs of high-ampli-tude spike, and-slow-wave dis-charges only in P7–13	Scantlebury et al. (2010)
	At P3 DOX+LPS At P5 PCPA		At P9–P20 other seizure types in 67 % (wild running, clonic seizures, behavioral arrest)					

TBI – parasagittal FPI

In vitro	Rat, P32–35, Spraque-Dawley, cortical slice	Cortical hyperexcit-ability, 8–10 weeks post-TBI	–	–	–	–	–	D'Ambrosio et al. [24]

(continued)

Table 1 (continued)

Model	Species, age, strain, preparation	Seizure susceptibility in vitro and/or in vivo	Epilepsy					Reference
			Animals with epilepsy (%)	Latency to spontaneous sz	Sz frequency	Sz duration (s)	Epileptiform spiking or EDs in EEG	
In vivo	Rat, P32–P35, Spraque-Dawley	n.d.	100 % (follow-up: 7 months)	~2 weeks	Up to 7 seizures/h	Ictal episodes ≤10 s (up to 99 s)	n.d.	D'Ambrosio et al. [24, 25]
TBI – lateral FPI								
In vivo	Rat, P19, Spraque-Dawley	No change in PTZ seizure threshold, 20 weeks post-TBI	0 % (behavioral observation)	n.d.	n.d.	n.d.	n.d.	Gurkoff et al. [39]
	Rat, P21–22, Wistar	Increased susceptibility to kainate-induced seizures, 6 week post-TBI	n.d.	n.d.	n.d.	n.d.	n.d.	Echegoyen et al. [32]
TBI – CCI								
In vitro	Rat, P24, Spraque-Dawley, cortical slice	Evoked (7–9 day post-TBI) and spontaneous epileptiform activity (14–16 day post-TBI)	–	–	–	–	–	Yang et al. (2010)

In vivo	Rat, P16–P18, Spraque-Dawley	Unchanged threshold for tonic hindlimb extension or minimal clonic seizures in electroconvulsive seizure threshold test, testing on P34–P40 Reduced threshold for minimal clonic seizures, testing on P60–P63	n.d.	n.d.	n.d.	n.d.	n.d.	Statler et al. [108]
	Rat, P17, Spraque-Dawley	n.d.	1 of 8 (13 %) (follow-up: 11 months)	n.d.	n.d.	45–60 s	88 % had epileptiform spiking	Statler et al. [109]

Only the data collected at least 1 week post-injury are included

Abbreviations: *CCI* controlled cortical impact, *ECS* electroconvulsive shock, *DOX/LPS/PCPA* doxorubicin, lipopolysaccharide, p-chlorophenylalanine, *FPI* fluid-percussion injury, *n.d.* no data, *sz* seizure, *P* postnatal day, *PPS* perforant path stimulation, *PTZ* pentylenetetrazol, *TBI* traumatic brain injury

recordings for seizure detection after administration of a high dose (170–380 mg/kg) of pilocarpine at P7 or older. Animals were observed for 3 months, and the occurrence of convulsive seizures was detected in a subpopulation of animals with SE at P18–P24, but not earlier. Interestingly, the proportion of animals that developed convulsive seizures increased with age at the time of SE induction. With video-EEG monitoring the development of epilepsy could already be demonstrated in animals that experienced SE in the second week of their life. For example, in a lithium-pilocarpine model, video-EEG monitoring demonstrated the development of epilepsy in a subpopulation of rats with SE as early as at P10 [111] or at P12 [61]. In these animals, unprovoked seizures monitored from 1 week to 1 month for up to 5 months after SE were subclinical nonconvulsive seizures with minor behavioral manifestations, including behavioral arrest and automatisms. Convulsive spontaneous seizures were never detected over the 1-year post-SE follow-up period (Kubova, in preparation). In P15 rats, lithium-pilocarpine-induced SE led to the development of spontaneous convulsive seizures within 4 months post-SE [97]. These data show that rather than resistance of the immature brain to SE-induced epilepsy, there is a substantial age-related difference in the semiology of SE-induced spontaneous seizures, and detection of subclinical seizures has been a key for this conclusion. One caveat in data interpretation relates to the difficulties in comparing the severity of SE and the extent of network activation during SE in different age groups.

In addition to the difficulties in detecting nonconvulsive seizures in rodents without EEG monitoring, the long latency period between SE and the onset of spontaneous seizures in immature animals compared to that for adult animals may have also contributed to the belief that SE is not able to trigger epileptogenesis in the immature brain. In adult animals, spontaneous recurrent seizures usually appear within a few days or a few weeks after SE. In rats with lithium-pilocarpine-induced SE at P12, a 1-week continuous video-EEG monitoring of animals at 3 months post-SE revealed spontaneous recurrent seizures in 25 % of the animals, at 5 months in 50 %, and at 7 months in 87.5 % ([61], Kubova, unpublished). In rats that experienced lithium-pilocarpine-induced SE at P10, 1-month continuous video-EEG monitoring started at 4 months post-SE revealed electrographic seizures in 55 % of animals (Suchomelova, unpublished).

Kainic Acid

Status epilepticus induced by systemic administration of kainic acid represents another frequently used model of acquired epilepsy. Systemic administration of kainic acid can produce SE in a reproducible way within the first 2 weeks of life [4, 15, 44]. In spite of its common use as a trigger of epileptogenesis in immature animals, the diagnosis of epilepsy after systemic kainate administration in adolescence or in adulthood has never been based on long-term video-EEG monitoring. Using intermittent video monitoring without EEG, Stafstrom and collaborators [106] detected spontaneous seizures in a subpopulation of rats when SE was induced with kainate at P20. Interestingly, no behavioral seizures were observed in animals with SE at a younger age.

Multiple Episodes of Chemically Induced SE

To induce neuropathological and functional changes in the developing brain by long-lasting epileptiform activity, some authors have triggered multiple episodes of SE. In one study only, however, spontaneous seizures were detected in parallel with behavioral deficits. Santos and collaborators [99] exposed P7–P9 animals to three episodes of pilocarpine-induced SE and, using extensive long-term video-EEG monitoring at 1–3 months post-SE (24 h/day for 30 days), they detected subclinical electrographic epileptiform activity, including epileptiform discharges characterized by frequent and continuous interictal spiking and polyspiking activity in the hippocampus or the neocortex, and in some cases the emergence of sudden rhythmic high-amplitude sustained discharges resembling electrographic seizures as well. They also reported spontaneous behavioral seizures in a small percentage of animals.

Other Approaches

In addition to systemic administration of chemoconvulsants as summarized above, many convulsants, particularly excitatory amino acid agonists, have been administered intracerebrally to trigger SE. A typical site of injection is either into a limbic structure like the amygdala or hippocampus, or into the cerebral ventricles. These models differ substantially from models of SE induced by systemic drug administration in terms of their neuropathological and functional sequelae, as they reflect the combination of the direct neurotoxic effects of the drug as well as the damaging effects of SE. Leite and collaborators [69] injected kainate unilaterally into the hippocampus in P7–P30 animals and monitored the rats with EEG for up to 8 months after SE. They found epileptiform activity and electrographic seizures in animals in all age groups, and a subpopulation of animals developed behavioral seizures. Neuropathology was highly dependent on age at the time of the kainate injection. The authors concluded that the model design could serve as a model of focal onset of seizures.

According to the "two-hit" hypothesis, two successive etiologies must work together to trigger neuropathological changes, epileptogenesis, and other functional impairments. The two-hit approach is relatively rarely used to model conditions that are commonly seen in patients with epilepsy. However, even the few data available provide evidence of a significant role of concomitant factors for the severity of consequences resulting from early-life SE. The lipopolysaccharide (LPS)-induced inflammatory response during lithium-pilocarpine-induced SE aggravated epileptogenesis in P14 rats [7]. Video-EEG monitoring (24 h/day for 6 days) performed 30 days after SE demonstrated that animals with inflammation developed convulsive seizures (stage 3–4), whereas only stage 1–2 seizures were detected in animals without inflammation. Increases in seizure frequency and severity (stage 3–4 compared to stage 1–2 seen in normothermic animals) were also observed in P10 rats that were exposed to hyperthermia (core temperature 39–40 °C) during lithium-pilocarpine-induced SE when assessed at 4 months post-SE [111].

Electrically Induced SE

The use of electrical stimulation as a trigger for SE provides a tool to avoid the direct toxic effects of chemoconvulsants. However, in immature rodents these studies are technically challenging. For example, fixing the electrode headset to the skull is difficult, particularly for the longer periods of time that would be needed for the follow-up of epileptogenesis. After-discharges can be induced at P7 and later, but SE can be triggered no earlier than during the third week of life. Still, some work with electrical stimulation has been done, particularly in juvenile rodents.

Electrical stimulation via perforant path stimulation (PPS) results in self-sustained SE in P21 rats, but not in younger rats. Spontaneous seizures have been detected only sporadically after PPS [98]. Detection of spontaneous seizures has, however, relied mostly on video monitoring, and only animals exhibiting spontaneous convulsive seizures have been subjected for further EEG recording.

Hyperthermia-Induced Experimental Febrile Seizures

In humans, prolonged febrile seizures or febrile SE presents a risk factor for the development of temporal lobe epilepsy later in life [113]. Under experimental conditions, *hyperthermic seizures* are generated by increasing body temperature in healthy immature animals. In P10 rats, a core temperature of approximately 40–41 °C lasting 24 min can trigger the development of spontaneous seizures in 40 % of rats over a 3–6-month follow-up period. Moreover, the majority of animals show epileptiform interictal activity [29]. In P11 rats, a core temperature of 39.5–41 °C lasting an average of 64 min results in SE, and increases the severity and duration of subsequent spontaneous seizures as compared to spontaneous seizures triggered by hyperthermic seizures in P10 rats [29]. It was calculated that P10 rats with hyperthermic seizures lasting 24 min had a 35 % probability of developing epilepsy, whereas in P11 rats that experienced hyperthermia-induced SE that lasted for about 64 min, the probability was 45 % [30]. It should be noted that Scantlebury et al. [100] induced hyperthermic seizures lasting for 20 min in rats at P10 but could not detect any spontaneous seizures 5.5 months after the initial insult, using EEG monitoring (20 min/day for 4–5 days) on rats at the same age as those of Dubé and colleagues [30]. One apparent explanation for this relates to the monitoring paradigm, as Dube et al. [29] monitored for 5 h/night at least five times between P90 and P180 and for 24 h twice a week or 48 h once a week [30].

Hypoxic-Ischemic Brain Damage (Models of Stroke)

In models of SE, the prolonged seizure activity initiates molecular and cellular cascades that trigger epileptogenesis. In models of hypoxic-ischemic brain damage, mechanisms other than intense seizure activity are believed to be responsible for the initial injury.

Ligation of the Common Carotid Artery

Studies on epileptogenesis after early hypoxic-ischemic insults are still limited. However, permanent ligation of the right common carotid artery in P7 rats followed by 120 min of exposure to hypoxia resulted in spontaneous convulsive seizures at 7–24 months post-injury in 40 % of rats [120]. Romijn et al. [94] induced hypoxic-ischemic injury in P12–P13 rats and found that a subpopulation of animals developed spontaneous electrographic seizures at 2.5 months post-injury. Interestingly, no convulsive seizures were detected. This discrepancy can be explained by the progressive nature of epilepsy in this model. Kadam and collaborators [53] demonstrated a remarkable increase in the severity of behavioral seizures after 3 months post-injury, suggesting that latency from injury to subclinical seizures is shorter than that to convulsive seizures.

Endothelin-1 Injection in the Hippocampus

Another method to trigger epileptogenesis by an ischemic lesion is to inject 20–40 pmol endothelin-1 (ET-1) unilaterally in the hippocampus. This results in focal ischemia and epileptogenesis in up to 91 % of P12 and P25 rats [75]. In concordance with the study by Romijn et al. [94], only nonconvulsive electrographic seizures were demonstrated in P12 and P25 animals 3 months after ET-1 [75]. As later intervals were not studied, it remains to be explored whether convulsive unprovoked seizures would appear after a longer latency.

Prolonged Hypoxia

There is a developmental window for increased susceptibility to hypoxia-induced seizures in rodents. The most severe seizures can be induced in P10–P12 rats [49, 50]. Consequently, when P10 rats were exposed to 15 min of hypoxia (4–7 % of O_2), video-EEG monitoring of P60–P80 rats revealed electrographic seizures in 94 % of these rats [92].

Early Seizures After Ischemia or Stroke

In humans, *early* seizures (<7 days post-stroke) can be detected in a subpopulation of patients with hypoxic-ischemic brain injury. They tend to be more frequent in infants and children than in adults [122]. These seizures should not be confused with late seizures (>1 week post-injury) as they more likely reflect the severity of the brain damage rather than a result of the epileptogenic process.

In rodents, the development of early seizures was described in a model of common carotid ligation combined with exposure to a reduced oxygen level in P12 mice [22]. In the ET-1 model of focal ischemia, early seizures were detected in both P12 and P25 rats within 24 h after infusion (video-EEG recording performed for 100 min after ET-1 infusion and repeated 22 h later). During the first monitoring period, seizures were convulsive (clonic movements, barrel rolling), with a frequency of around six (P12) or three (P25) seizures per 100 min and an average duration of around 30 s in both age groups. At 22 h later, only nonconvulsive seizures were detected and they tended to be shorter and less frequent [75, 114]. In both age groups, there was also a positive correlation between the severity of acute damage at 24 h post-ET-1 injection, total seizure duration (i.e., total duration of early seizures registered during the first 100 min after the injection of ET-1), and the severity of behavioral seizures.

The developmental aspects of early post-injury seizures were also studied in a model of global hypoxia. In newborn piglets, hypoxia (4 % of O_2 for 30 min combined with 10 min of hypotension) induced both convulsive (in 46 % of animals) and subclinical (29 % of animals) seizures. Subclinical seizures were detected using EEG monitoring (2 h/day for 3 days after the insult). Clinical seizures were defined as myoclonic jerks, clonic movements, tonic posture, and rhythmic pathological movements (cycling) [8]. The long-term consequences of these seizures were not studied.

Traumatic Brain Injury

Traumatic brain injury (TBI) is defined as an alteration in brain function, or other evidence of brain pathology, caused by an external force [77]. In children, the risk of epilepsy is increased even after a mild TBI (2.2-fold), and the risk continues to be elevated for 10 years after the TBI. Moreover, the risk of epilepsy increases with age after mild or severe injury and is especially high among people older than 15 years of age [19]. Experimental studies on pediatric TBI are scarce, and even fewer studies are available on post-traumatic epilepsy in immature rats.

Parasagittal Fluid-Percussion Injury (FPI)

D'Ambrosio and colleagues [24, 25] recently induced rostral parasagittal FPI in juvenile male Sprague-Dawley rats at postnatal day 32–35. The center of the 3-mm-diameter burr hole was located 2 mm posterior to the bregma and 3 mm lateral to the midline. A fluid pressure pulse of 3.75–4 atm was applied. Intermittent extended video-electrocorticography (EcoG) with epidural electrodes demonstrated partial seizures originating in the neocortex proximal to the lesion site with or without secondary generalization. The majority (60 %) of animals displayed electrographic epileptiform activity within the first 2 weeks post-injury. Epileptiform activity was present in 100 % of animals 9 weeks after injury. Ictal EcoG events were categorized into three different grades: grade 1 activity originating from the cortical lesion focus and limited to it, grade 2 activity originating from the focus with subsequent spread, and grade 3 activity (generalized) starting simultaneously in several channels. Ictal episodes consisted of 7–10-Hz rhythmical spike-wave discharges of up to 10-s duration with abrupt onset and end. During ictal discharges, injured animals typically demonstrated behavioral arrest that was sometimes followed by facial automatisms, myoclonus, or "ictal atonia." Tonic-clonic behavioral seizures or complete electrographic seizures have not been reported. In vitro local field potential recordings demonstrated persistent hyperexcitability of the neocortex at the site and around the lesion that was associated with increased glial reactivity. In a 7-month follow-up study, ictal-like episodes originating in the hippocampus were reported, which gradually increased in frequency, suggesting that the ictal focus moved from the frontoparietal cortex (at or near the site of injury) to the temporal lobe. Interestingly, idiopathic seizures were observed in 33 % of the control rat population at 27–28 weeks post-injury. Cresyl violet and glial fibrillary acidic protein (GFAP) staining indicated that early pathologic changes were confined to the lesioned cortex and thalamus. Changes included neuronal loss, areas of calcification, and reactive gliosis. In a chronic follow-up study, atrophy of the CA1 and CA3 subfields of the hippocampus ipsilateral to the injury site was also reported.

Lateral Fluid-Percussion Injury (FPI)

Gurkoff et al. [39] induced TBI by using lateral FPI at P19. None of the rats displayed any convulsive seizure activity over the 20-week follow-up period. Also, there was no change in seizure threshold for PTZ-induced seizures. Rats had hardly any neurodegeneration in the hilus, CA1, or CA2 ipsilaterally or contralaterally. Also, the average density of mossy fiber sprouting did not differ from that in controls, even though a few animals had abnormal sprouting. Echegoyen et al. [32] induced lateral FPI in P21–P22 rats. The animals showed increased susceptibility to kainate-induced seizures at 6 weeks post-TBI.

Controlled Cortical Impact (CCI)

The development of epilepsy was studied in immature (P17) Sprague-Dawley rats following CCI [108, 109]. Video-EEG monitoring was performed for 3 months (range 9–90 days), starting at 4–8 months post-injury. The majority (88 %) of injured rats exhibited epileptiform EEG activity in the form of isolated spikes. Generalized clonic seizures accompanied by an ictal electrographic pattern were observed in one of eight TBI animals, which had a total of four seizures lasting 45–60 s during the monitoring period. Latency to the first seizure was 260 days and seizures appeared to be organized in a cluster. This preliminary study suggests that CCI during immaturity represents a potential model for pediatric PTE. Interestingly, the PTE model induced by CCI in immature rats demonstrated features similar to those described in lateral FPI in adult rats [54], such as relatively low prevalence of PTE and low seizure frequency, long latency period, and seizure clustering. Further investigations with a more intensive EEG monitoring paradigm, larger sample sizes, and a greater number of electrodes are warranted to establish the clinical relevance of this model.

Models of Age-Related Syndromes or Epilepsies

Catastrophic childhood epilepsies such as infantile spasms and Lennox-Gastaut syndrome are examples of serious neurological disorders in childhood because of their intractability to conventionally available antiepileptic drugs and their association with cognitive decline. Animal models of these specific age-related syndromes and epilepsies are of particular interest because they would provide the opportunity to test syndrome-specific treatment strategies. Despite this great clinical importance, few models are available. In fact, there are only two models for infantile spasms proposed so far. In a subpopulation of P10–P12 rats, continual intracortical or intrahippocampal infusion of tetrodotoxin (TTX) lasting 4 weeks [67] resulted in the development of spasm-like seizures in about 30 % of the animals. Seizures continued for days after the end of infusion. In some animals, spasms were observed up to 2 months after TTX infusion. So far, there are no data on the psychomotor development of affected animals or on the efficacy of antiepileptic drugs against spasm-like seizures in this model.

A multiple-hit model was recently proposed by Scantlebury and collaborators (2010). Animals were subjected to an intracerebral injection of LPS and doxorubicin at P3. Two days later (P5) they received an intraperitoneal injection of p-chlorophenylalanine. Spasm-like seizures appeared in all animals. In 67 % of animals between P9 and P20, other seizure types (tonic seizures, wild running, behavioral arrest) were also observed. In addition to spontaneous seizures, the affected animals exhibited retardation of psychomotor development. Vigabatrin but not ACTH suppressed the spasms. However, the effect of vigabatrin was transient.

In both models of infantile spasms, spontaneous seizures occurred after an insult or drug infusion, at least for a limited period of time. Further studies are needed to explore their relevance to the human syndrome.

Seizure Susceptibility and the Risk of Epilepsy After Brain Insults in the Immature Brain

Whether an increase in seizure susceptibility after brain insults can be considered as a biomarker for later development of epilepsy is a major research challenge, particularly for studies that investigate novel antiepileptogenic treatments.

Several studies have suggested that SE early in life can change seizure susceptibility in adulthood, even without the development of epilepsy. Moreover, the results, even though inconclusive, suggest that the effects of SE on seizure susceptibility are age-related. For example, kainate-induced SE at P1–P14 resulted in an enhanced paired-pulse inhibition in the dentate gyrus and reduced kindling susceptibility 3 months later [74]. However, SE at P21 and P24 resulted in a chronic decrease in $GABA_A$-dependent paired-pulse inhibition in the dentate gyrus [74, 98]. Another study showed that kainate-induced SE at P27 increased the susceptibility to hippocampal kindling at 3 days and 3 months post-SE. However, Holmes and Thompson [46] reported that in animals with kainate-induced SE at P12 or P18, the rate of kindling remained unchanged when assessed at P15, P21, and P30. Moreover, in rats with SE induced with lithium-pilocarpine at P12 or P25, the excitability of the sensorimotor cortex was decreased rather than increased within the first month after the insult [115].

Early hyperthermic seizures can also enhance hippocampal excitability and seizure susceptibility later in life. In P10–P11 rats, prolonged hyperthermic seizures (core temperature around 41°C) lasting for 20–30 min reduced the threshold for kainate-induced seizures in vivo 2 months later, and enhanced limbic excitability in vitro already at 1 week post-insult in the absence of any spontaneous recurrent seizures [28]. Gulec and Noyan [38] induced multiple hyperthermic seizures lasting for 20 min in P25 rats by immersing the animals in warm water (45 °C) until the first seizure appeared (2–4 min) once a day every second day for up to eight times. When assessed at P60–P70, rats showed enhanced susceptibility to pilocarpine-induced SE. Also, rats exposed to hyperthermic seizures (ambient temperature 45°C) lasting for 20 min at P30 exhibited enhanced susceptibility to kainate-induced seizures 2 months later [124].

Both global hypoxia and hypoxia-ischemia at an early age can also modify the susceptibility to or characteristics of induced seizures at adolescence or adulthood. Moreover, data from models of global hypoxia suggest that changes in seizure susceptibility are dependent on the severity of the ischemic-hypoxic insult and the age at the time of insult. For example, P10 rats exposed to asphyxia (100 % N_2) exhibited a long-term increase in susceptibility to PTZ and kindling compared to controls [18, 76]. Animals that underwent global hypoxia (3–4 % O_2) at P10 also exhibited increased susceptibility to PTZ and flurothyl-induced seizures, as well as to amygdaloid kindling later in life [49–51]. In contrast, there was no difference in the rate of kindling or susceptibility to flurothyl-induced seizures between rats that were exposed to mild hypoxia (6 % O_2) at P1 or P10 and tested at the fourth week of life [80]. Also, an 8-h exposure of P25 rats to hypobaric hypoxia (simulated altitude of 7,000 m), which is another model of mild hypoxia, resulted only in a transiently increased severity of PTZ-induced seizures at 3 days post-insult but not at 1 or 7 days after insult [62].

Induction of focal ischemia at P7 by unilateral occlusion of the carotid artery followed by 2 h of hypoxia resulted in a transient increase in seizure susceptibility to bicuculline-induced seizures. The maximum increase in seizure susceptibility was found at 24 h post-insult. When tested at shorter or longer intervals, seizure severity was rather suppressed than increased [14]. Holmes and Weber [45] demonstrated that moderate to severe hypoxia-ischemia induced by carotid ligation at P13 or at P28 inhibited the development of generalized seizures when animals were exposed to an amygdala kindling paradigm 2 days after the insult. Taken together, these available data suggest that hypoxic-ischemic insults suppress late seizure susceptibility in the majority of animals, even if the insult eventually results in the development of epilepsy. However, longer-term studies are necessary to assess changes in seizure susceptibility and to find out whether and how the susceptibility to induced seizures relates to ongoing epileptogenesis.

Transcriptomics, Epigenetics, MicroRNAs, Proteomics, and Metabolomics After Acquired Epileptogenic Injuries in the Immature Brain

Alterations in gene expression in acquired pediatric epilepsy have not been studied as much as they have in adult epilepsy [73, 88]. For example, to the best of our knowledge, there are only three datasets derived from microarray analyses that describe gene expression following SE and there is one dataset following hypoxia-ischemia in juvenile animals [3, 42, 43, 66, 121], while several datasets are available for adult epilepsy models and human tissue [73, 88].

Akahoshi et al. [3] studied changes in gene expression levels in the neocortex and hippocampus 7 days after repeated intraperitoneal injections of kainic acid in P23 mice. Although the authors focused on only cathepsin S, the supplementary data provided on the microarray analysis show that altogether 34 genes were upregulated and 39 downregulated in either the neocortex or the hippocampus. Our analysis of this dataset using Biological Process Gene Ontology Terms in the David Functional Annotation Tool (http://david.abcc.ncifcrf.gov; [26, 47]) revealed that the products of regulated genes participate in immune response, phosphorylation, regulation of cell death, angiogenesis, regulation of transcription, or synaptic transmission.

Lauren et al. [66] performed a microarray analysis of gene expression in the CA1 area of the hippocampus 7 days after intraperitoneal injection of kainic acid in P21 rats. As many as 1,592 genes were differentially expressed in kainic acid-treated animals compared to controls. Genes involved in oxidative phosphorylation, long-term potentiation, Ca^{2+} homeostasis, gliosis, inflammation, and GABAergic transmissions had altered expression levels. Interestingly, only upregulation of cathepsin S and apolipoprotein E and downregulation of calbindin 1 mRNA expression were detected in studies by Akahosi et al. [3] and Lauren et al. [65].

The third microarray dataset describes changes in gene expression at earlier time points as well, that is, at 1–240 h following intraperitoneal injection of kainic acid in P15 or P30 rats [121]. This dataset was used to evaluate the influence of SE on neuropeptides and their receptors. More changes were observed in older than in younger animals. Administration of kainic acid at P15 evoked a transient induction of mRNA expression of thyrotrophin-releasing hormone (TRH), neuropeptide Y (NPY), cortistatin (CST), corticotropin-releasing hormone (CRH), corticotropin-releasing hormone binding protein (CRH-BP), and trachikinin (Tac1). The regulation was most prominent at 6–24 h after SE [121].

Hedtjarn and co-workers performed an extensive analysis of the transcriptome in P9 mice that were exposed to common carotid artery ligation followed by hypoxia [42, 43]. Gene expression was studied at 2, 8, 24, and 72 h after hypoxia-ischemia in the cortex, hippocampus, thalamus, and striatum. Levels of expression were compared between ipsilateral and contralateral hemispheres and to those in control animals. Altogether, 283 genes were upregulated and 60 were downregulated. Regulated genes were related to transcription, stress response and apoptosis, growth, signal transduction, cell cycle, cytoskeleton function, transport, and ion transport and metabolism. Interestingly, genes involved in the regulation of transcription or metabolism were frequently upregulated, while genes involved in ion or vesicular transport and signal transduction were frequently downregulated [42, 43]. A large functional gene category of regulated genes detected in the same dataset included genes involved in the inflammatory response [42, 43]. As many as 144 upregulated and 4 downregulated genes could be assigned to this functional category, including chemokines, complement, genes expressed by leukocytes and macrophages, genes coding proteins involved in interferon action, MHC, and adhesion proteins [42, 43].

In addition to global analyses of gene expression, data on changes in mRNA expression of selected genes detected by in situ hybridization or PCR are also available. Such genes were usually selected for the study on the basis of previous knowledge, carrying a presumed role in functional or structural plasticity or in response to damage (Table 2).

Although there are data on altered gene expression following epileptogenic stimuli in young animals for a substantial number of genes, there is little overlap between different studies. Each of the global transcriptome studies resulted in detection of alterations of a different ensemble of genes, while studies using a gene-by-gene approach provided only limited information concerning single genes. When the functions of genes regulated by an epileptogenic insult are considered, the most affected functional groups of genes are those involved in cell death, inflammation and immune response, signal transduction, and regulation of transcription or ion transport. This resembles the alterations in the transcriptome response to brain-damaging insults in the adult brain [73, 88].

So far, there are no published reports on epigenetics, microRNAs, proteomics, metabolomics, or lipidomics during epileptogenesis in immature animals, even though these data would be of great importance considering the major effects of these regulatory systems on gene transcription and translation. Also, data on proteomics or metabolomics analyses are not available. Consequently, as summarized in Table 3, attempts to prevent epileptogenesis in the immature brain have not really benefitted from molecular analyses of epileptogenic tissue but rather have used traditional approaches by trying to prevent epileptogenesis with available antiepileptic drugs, without any success.

Table 2 Alterations in mRNA expression in the immature brain in models of acquired pediatric epilepsy studied with PCR, Northern blot, or in situ hybridization

Gene symbol	Description	Animal model	Age	Observation	Source
GABRA1	Gamma-aminobutyric acid (GABA) A receptor, alpha 1	SE with lithium-pilocarpine	P10	↑ Dentate gyrus, adult	Zhang et al. [123]
		SE with kainic acid	P9	↓ CA3, 1 week	Lauren et al. [65]
GABRA4	Gamma-aminobutyric acid (GABA) A receptor, alpha 4	SE with kainic acid	P9	↓ Dentate gyrus, 6 h	Lauren et al. [65]
GABRB1	Gamma-aminobutyric acid (GABA) A receptor, beta 1	SE with kainic acid	P9	↑ CA1, 6 h	Lauren et al. [65]
GABRB3	Gamma-aminobutyric acid (GABA) A receptor, beta 3	SE with kainic acid	P9	↑ CA1, 1 week	Lauren et al. [65]
GABG1	Gamma-aminobutyric acid (GABA) A receptor, gamma 1	SE with kainic acid	P9	↓ CA3c, 6 h; ↓ CA1, 6 h; ↓ dentate gyrus, 3days	Lauren et al. [65]
GABG2	Gamma-aminobutyric acid (GABA) A receptor, gamma 2	SE with kainic acid	P9	↓ CA3c, 6 h, 3days; ↓ CA1, 6 h, 3days; ↓ dentate gyrus, 6 h, 3days	Lauren et al. [65]
SLC12A2	Solute carrier family 12 (sodium/potassium/chloride transporters), member 2, (NKCC1)	Cortical freeze-lesion	P0	↑ Surrounding lesion, 4days	Shimizu-Okabe et al. [104]
SLC12A5	Solute carrier family 12 (potassium/chloride transporter), member 5, (KCC2)	Cortical freeze-lesion	P0	↓ Surrounding lesion, 4days	Shimizu-Okabe et al. [104]
HCN1	Hyperpolarization activated cyclic nucleotide-gated potassium channel 1	Hyperthermia-induced experimental febrile seizures		↓ CA1 up to 3 months	Brewster et al. [11]

HCN2	Hyperpolarization activated cyclic nucleotide-gated potassium channel 2	Hyperthermia-induced experimental febrile seizures	P10–P11	↑ CA1 and CA3	Brewster et al. [11]
GRIA1	Glutamate receptor, ionotropic, AMPA 1 (Glur1)	SE with kainic acid	P14	↑ Dentate gyrus	Friedman et al. [34]
GRIA2	Glutamate receptor, ionotropic, AMPA 2 (Glur2)	SE with kainic acid	P14	↑ Dentate gyrus	Friedman et al. [34]
		Hypoxia-ischemia	P10	↓ Neocortex and hippocampus, 2days	Sanchez et al. [96]
		Hypoxia-induced seizures	P10–P12	↓ Neocortex and hippocampus, 48 h	Sanchez et al. [96]
		SE with lithium-pilocarpine	P20	↑ Dentate gyrus, 2 weeks	Porter et al. [91]
GRIA3	Glutamate receptor, ion-otrophic, AMPA 3 (Glur3)	SE with lithium-pilocarpine		↓ Dentate gyrus, 2 weeks	Porter et al. [91]
GRIK2	Glutamate receptor, ionotropic, kainate 2 (Glur6)	SE with lithium-pilocarpine		↓ Dentate gyrus, 2 weeks	Porter et al. [91]
GRIK5	Glutamate receptor, ionotropic, kainate 5	SE with lithium-pilocarpine		↑ Dentate gyrus, 2 weeks	Porter et al. [91]
GRM2	Glutamate receptor, metabotro-pic 2 (mGlur2)	SE with kainic acid	P10	↓ Dentate gyrus, 1 day	Aronica et al. [6]
GRM4	Glutamate receptor, metabotro-pic 4 (mGlur4)	SE with kainic acid	P10	↑ CA3, 1 day	Aronica et al. [6]
SLC38A1	Solute carrier family 38, member 1 (SNAT1)	Hypoxia-ischemia	P7	↓ Both hemispheres, 1 h	Leibovici et al. [68]
Htr5b	5-Hydroxytryptamine (serotonin) receptor 5B	SE with kainic acid	P21	↓ Hippocampus, 10 days	Koh et al. [57]
DRD1	Dopamine receptor D1	Hypoxia-ischemia	P7	↓ Striatum, 2–21 days	Filloux et al. [33]
DRD2	Dopamine receptor D2	Hypoxia-ischemia	P7	↓ Striatum up to 2 h	Filloux et al. [33]
		Hypoxia-ischemia	P7	↓ Striatum, 24 h	Cantagrel et al. [13]

(continued)

Table 2 (continued)

Gene symbol	Description	Animal model	Age	Observation	Source
BDNF	Brain-derived neurotrophic factor	SE with lithium-pilocarpine	P7, P12	↑ Hippocampus, piriform and entorhinal cortex, 2–4 h	Kornblum et al. [58]
		SE with kainic acid	P7	↑ CA3	Kornblum et al. [58]
		SE with kainic acid	P13, P21	↑ Hippocampus	Dugich-Djordjevic et al. [31]
IGF-BP 2	Insulin-like growth factor binding protein 2	Hypoxia-ischemia	P21	↑ CA1/CA3 and thalamus at 3 days; thalamus and infarct in lateral-parietal cortex at 5 days	Klempt et al. [55]
SYP	Synaptophysin	SE with lithium-pilocarpine	P21	↑ Piriform and entorhinal cortex	Hanaya et al. [41]
TP53	Tumor protein p53 (p53)	SE with lithium-pilocarpine	P15 and P21	↑ Hippocamus, piriform cortex, amygdale,thalamus, 8 h	Tan et al. [112]
HSPA1A	Heat shock 70 kDa protein 1A (HSP72)	Hypoxia-ischemia	P7	↑ Ipsilateral hemisphere, 2 h; cortex, CA1–CA3, 24 h	Kobayashi and Welsh [56]
HSPA1	Heat shock 70 kDa protein (HSP70)	SE with kainic acid	P21	↑ Hippocampus 4–16 h	Little et al. [71]
		Hypoxia-ischemia	P7	↑ Ipsilateral hemisphere, 1–24 h	Gubits et al. [37]
		Hypoxia-ischemia	P7	↑ Ipsilateral hemisphere, 2 h, 24 h	Kobayashi and Welsh [56]
		Hypoxia-ischemia	P7	↑ Cortex, hippocampus, striatum 10 min-24 h	Munell et al. [81]
HSPA5	Heat shock 70 kDa protein 5 (glucose-regulated protein, 78 kDa, Grp78)	SE with kainic acid	P14, P21	↑ Hippocampus 4–8 h, neocortex 4–16 h	Little et al. [71]
HSP90B	Heat shock protein 90 kDa beta (Grp94)	SE with kainic acid	P7, P14, P21	↑ CA3, neocortex, 16 h ↑ CA1, 4–8 h, dentate gyrus neocortex, for up to 16 h	Little et al. [71]
BAX	BCL2-associated X protein	Hypoxia-ischemia	P7	↑ Ipsilateral hemisphere, 4 h, 12 h	Kumral et al. [64]

HRK	Harakiri, BCL2 interacting protein (DP5)	Hypoxia-ischemia	P7	↑ Ipsilateral hemisphere, 4 h, 12 h	Kumral et al. [64]
GFAP	Glial fibrillary acidic protein	Hypoxia-ischemia	P7	↑ Ipsilateral forebrain, 18 and 34 h	Gubits et al. [37]
		Hypoxia-ischemia	P7	↑ Ipsilateral cortex, 1–14days	Burtrum and Silverstein [12]
TNF	Tumor necrosis factor (TNF-alpha)	SE with kainic acid	P21	↑ Hippocampus, 4 h	Rizzi et al. [93]
		Hypoxia-ischemia	P7	↑ ipsilateral hemisphere, 1–24 h	Bona et al. [10]
Il6	Interleukin 6 (interferon, beta 2)	SE with kainic acid	P21	↑ hippocampus, 4 h	Rizzi et al. [93]
		Hypoxia-ischemia	P7	↑ Hemisphere, 3–6 h	Hagberg et al. [40]
Il1B	Interleukin 1 beta	SE with kainic acid	P15, P21	↑ Hippocampus, 4 h	Rizzi et al. [93]
		Hypoxia-ischemia	P7	↑ Hemisphere, 3–6 h	Hagberg et al. [40]
		Hypoxia-ischemia	P7	↑ Ipsilateral hemisphere, 0–12 h	Bona et al. [10]
IL1R1	Interleukin 1 beta (IL1Ra)	SE with kainic acid	P21	↑ Hippocampus, 4 h	Rizzi et al. [93]
Il10	Interleukin 10	Hypoxia-ischemia	P7	↓ Ipsilateral hemisphere, 0–1 h, 14 days	Kremlev et al. [60]
CXCL1	Chemokine (C-X-C motif) ligand 1 (GRO1)	Hypoxia-ischemia	P7	↑ Ipsilateral hemisphere, 6–24 h	Bona et al. [10]
CCl2	Chemokine (C-C motif) ligand 2 (MCP-1)	Hypoxia-ischemia	P7	↑ Ipsilateral hemisphere, 4–24 h	Ivacko et al. [48]
CCL3	Chemokine (C-C motif) ligand 3 (MIP-1-alpha)	Hypoxia-ischemia	P7	↑ Ipsilateral hemisphere, 1–24 h	Kremlev et al. [60]
CCL4	Chemokine (C-C motif) ligand 4 (MIP-1-beta)	Hypoxia-ischemia	P7	↑ Ipsilateral hemisphere, 1–24 h	Bona et al. [10]
CXCL2	Chemokine (C-X-C motif) ligand 3 (GRO3)	Hypoxia-ischemia	P7	↑ Ipsilateral hemisphere, 0–24 h	Bona et al. [10]
CCL5	Chemokine (C-C motif) ligand 5 (RANTES)	Hypoxia-ischemia	P7	↑ Ipsilateral hemisphere, 24 h and 14 days	Bona et al. [10]

(continued)

Table 2 (continued)

Gene symbol	Description	Animal model	Age	Observation	Source
CCR5	Chemokine (C-C motif) receptor 5	Hypoxia-ischemia	P7	↑ Ipsilateral hemisphere, 3–24 h	Kremlev et al. [60]
				↑ Ipsilateral hemisphere, 3–7 days	Cowell et al. [23]
CXCR3	Chemokine (C-X-C motif) receptor 3	Hypoxia-ischemia	P7	↑ Ipsilateral hemisphere, 3–24 h	Kremlev et al. [60]
LGALS3	Lectin, galactoside-binding, soluble 3 (galectin-3)	Hypoxia-ischemia	P9 mice	↑ Ipsilateral hemisphere, 8–72 h	Doverhag et al. [27]
PDGFB	Platelet-derived growth factor beta polypeptide	Hypoxia-ischemia	P7	↑ Ipsilateral and contralateral cortex, 3 h–7 days	Ohno et al. [85]
PDGFRA	Platelet-derived growth factor receptor alpha polypeptide	Hypoxia-ischemia	P7	↑ Ipsilateral cortex, 0.5–48 h	Morioka et al. [79]
EPOR	Erythropoietin receptor	Hypoxia-ischemia	P7	↑ Ipsilateral hemisphere 0–24 h	Spandou et al. [105]
FOS	FBJ murine osteosarcoma viral oncogene homolog (c-fos)	Hypoxia-ischemia	P7	↑ Both hemispheres, 2 h	Aden et al. [1]
				↑ Ipsilateral and contralateral forebrain, 1–3 h	Gubits et al. [37]
		Hypoxia-ischemia	P7	↑ Cortex, hippocampus, striatum 10 min–24 h	Munell et al. [81]
JUN	Jun proto-oncogene (c-jun)	Hypoxia-ischemia	P7	↑ Ipsilateral and contralateral forebrain, 1–3 h	Gubits et al. [37]
		Hypoxia-ischemia	P7	↑ Cortex, hippocampus, striatum 10 min–24 h	Munell et al. [81]
Nr4A1	Nuclear receptor subfamily 4, group A, member 1	Hypoxia-ischemia	P7	↑ Ipsilateral and contralateral forebrain, 1–3 h	Gubits et al. [37]
ERG1	Early growth response 1 (zif268)	Hypoxia-ischemia	P7	↑ Ipsilateral and contralateral forebrain, 1–3 h	Gubits et al. [37]
ZFP36	Zinc finger protein 36	Hypoxia-ischemia	P7	↑ Ipsilateral and contralateral forebrain, 1–3 h	Gubits et al. [37]

SLC2A1	Solute carrier family 2 (facilitated glucose transporter), member 1 (Glut1)	SE with pentylenetetrazol	P10 and P21	↑ All areas, 1–4 h	Nehlig et al. [83]
SLC2A3	Solute carrier family 2 (facilitated glucose transporter), member 3, (Glut3)	SE with pentylenetetrazol	P10 and P21	↑ All areas, 1–4 h	Nehlig et al. [83]
CLU	Clusterin	Hypoxia-ischemia	P21	↑ In and around hippocampal fissure 2–7 days; granule cell layer 6–24 h; CA3 6 h-3 days; cortex 2–7 days	Walton et al. [117]
RTN4	Reticulon 4 (NOGOA)	Hypoxia-ischemia	P7	↑ Ipsilateral cortex, 6–12 h	Wang et al. [118]
RTN4R	Reticulon 4 receptor (NgR)	Hypoxia-ischemia	P7	↑ Ipsilateral cortex, 6–12 h	Wang et al. [118]
ADORA1	Adenosine A1 receptor	Hypoxia-ischemia	P7	↓ Ipsilateral hemisphere, 0–2 h	Aden et al. [2]
ADORA2A	Adenosine A2a receptor	Hypoxia-ischemia	P7	↓ Ipsilateral hemisphere, 0–2 h	Aden et al. [2]
P2RX7	Purinergic receptor P2X, ligand-gated ion channel 7	Hypoxia-ischemia	P3	↓ Ipsilateral cortex, hippocampus, and subcortical white matter, 2 h	Wang et al. [119]

Table 3 A summary of antiepileptogenesis trials in different animal models of acquired pediatric epilepsy

AED	Model	Age[a]	Beginning of treatment	Duration of treatment	Effect on epileptogenesis	Disease modification (seizure characteristics and memory in epileptic animals)	Reference
Models of SE							
Felbamate	KA (i.p.)	P30	1 h after KA injection	1 dose	Seizure susceptibility (flurothyl) ±0	Seizures n.d. Memory impairment: ⇩	Chronopoulos et al. [20]
Gabapentin	Kainic acid	P36	24 h after the beginning of SE	P36–P75	Epileptogenesis ⇩ (?) during drug taper	Seizure characteristics: n.d. Memory impairment: ±0	Cilio et al. [21]
Lamotrigine	Li-pilocarpine	P12 P25	1 h after the beginning of SE	7 days	Epileptogenesis n.d.	Seizures ±0 Memory impairment: ⇩	Kubova H, personal communication
Phenobarbital	Kainic acid (i.p.)	P35	24 h after the beginning of SE	P36–P153	n.d. (?)	Seizure frequency ±0 Memory impairment: ⇧	Mikati et al. [78]
	Kainic acid (i.p.)	P35	24 h after the beginning of SE	P36–P75	±0 during drug taper (?)	Seizure frequency ±0 Memory impairment: ±0	Bolanos et al. [9]
Pregabalin	Li-pilocarpine	P21	20 min after pilocarpine	13 days	Epileptogenesis ±0 (?) Latency ⇧ (?)	Seizures: n.d. Memory impairment: n.d.	Andre et al. [5]
Topiramate	Neonatals seizures (flurothyl; 5/ day, total 25)	P0–P4	24 h after the last seizure	P6–P30	Epileptogenesis n.d.	Seizures: n.d. Memory impairment: ±0	Cha et al. [16]
	Li-pilocarpine	P20	10 min after beginning of SE	1 dose	Epileptogenesis ⇩	Seizure frequency ⇩ Interictal spikes ⇩ Memory impairment: n.d.	Suchomelova et al. [111]
	Li-pilocarpine	P28					

Valproate	Kainic acid	P35	24 h after the beginning of SE	P36–P75	⇩ During drug taper	No animals with spontaneous seizures Memory imapirment: ⇩	Bolanos et al. [9]
Hyperthermia-induced experimental febrile seizures							
SR141716A		P10	2 min after start of seizure induction	1 dose	Seizure susceptibility ⇩ at 1 week in vitro (electrical stimulation) and at 6 weeks in vivo (kainate)	n.a.	Chen et al. [17]
Models of TBI							
SR141716A	Lateral FPI	P21–P22	2 min post-TBI	1 dose	Seizure susceptibility ⇩	n.a.	Echegoyen et al. [32]

Abbreviations: *AED* antiepileptic drug, *HC* hippocampus, *n.d.* no data available, *n.a.* not applicable, ±0 no effect, ⇩ decrease in epileptogenesis or alleviation of the severity of epilepsy or memory impairment, (?) monitoring of the occurrence of spontaneous seizures was based on visual observation and counting of secondarily generalized behavioral seizures

[a]Age at the time of insult

Conclusions

Over recent years there has been a remarkable increase in the number of studies using long-term video-EEG monitoring in immature animals in models of acquired epileptogenesis. New models, for example, for infantile spasms have also been developed. Data from these studies have provided a more accurate insight into the process of epileptogenesis in different conditions, which could be expected to help develop the strategy of molecular analyses aimed at finding novel treatment targets and biomarkers to combat epileptogenesis in the immature brain. For example, there is quite consistent evidence from several laboratories that the developmental stage at the time of insult is critical for future outcome. Despite the availability of more accurate data on the clinical phenotype of epileptogenesis, a lack of transcriptional analyses and a complete lack of data on epigenetic and microRNA regulation of epileptogenesis in the immature brain is surprising. To be able to make evidence-based approaches to prevent epileptogenesis in the immature brain, better use of molecular data acquired in pediatric models is needed to avoid the situation whereby the antiepileptogenic treatments for pediatric epilepsies are derived from studies done in adults, as is the case in the development of antiepileptic drugs.

Proposals for the Future

The International League Against Epilepsy (ILAE) and The American Epilepsy Society (AES) have recently established a joint task force to improve the preclinical study designs used in investigating novel antiepileptogenic and antiepileptic drugs [36]. Studies dealing with the immature brain represent one dimension of the work. Beyond optimizing the study designs, there is a clear need to expand the methodological armamentarium, including animal models, particularly those that model catastrophic childhood epilepsies. There is also a need to develop more advanced miniature technologies for long-term video-EEG monitoring and analysis in small animals. Moreover, more systematic data on the molecular mechanisms and the regulation of transcription and translation in the immature brain during epileptogenesis are required. Despite many positive past achievements, more work remains to be done in order to be able to prevent epileptogenesis in children at risk, to monitor disease progression, and to evaluate treatment responses through using relevant biomarkers.

Acknowledgements This study was supported by the Academy of Finland (AP), The Sigrid Juselius Foundation (AP), CURE (AP), PMSE grant 888/N-ESF-EuroEPINOMICS/10/2011/0 (KL), statutory funds of the Nencki Institute (KL), grant Nos. P302/10/0971 and P304/12/G069 from the Grant Agency of the Czech Republic (HK), grant No. ME08045 from the Ministry of Education of the Czech Republic (HK), and by the long-term strategic development financing of the Institute of Physiology ASCR RVO:67985823 (HK).

References

1. Aden U, Bona E, Hagberg H, Fredholm BB (1994) Changes in c-fos mRNA in the neonatal rat brain following hypoxic ischemia. Neurosci Lett 180:91–95
2. Aden U, Lindstrom K, Bona E, Hagberg H, Fredholm BB (1994) Changes in adenosine receptors in the neonatal rat brain following hypoxic ischemia. Brain Res Mol Brain Res 23:354–358
3. Akahoshi N, Murashima YL, Himi T, Ishizaki Y, Ishii I (2007) Increased expression of the lysosomal protease cathepsin S in hippocampal microglia following kainate-induced seizures. Neurosci Lett 429:136–141
4. Albala BJ, Moshé SL, Okada R (1984) Kainic-acid-induced seizures: a developmental study. Brain Res 315:139–148
5. André V, Rigoulot MA, Koning E, Ferrandon A, Nehlig A (2003) Long-term pregabalin treatment protects basal cortices and delays the occurrence of spontaneous seizures in the lithium-pilocarpine model in the rat. Epilepsia 44(7):893–903
6. Aronica EM, Gorter JA, Paupard MC, Grooms SY, Bennett MV, Zukin RS (1997) Status epilepticus-induced alterations in metabotropic glutamate receptor expression in young and adult rats. J Neurosci 17:8588–8595
7. Auvin S, Mazarati A, Shin D, Sankar R (2010) Inflammation enhances epileptogenesis in the developing rat brain. Neurobiol Dis 40:303–310
8. Björkman ST, Miller SM, Rose SE, Burke C, Colditz PB (2010) Seizures are associated with brain injury severity in a neonatal model of hypoxia-ischemia. Neuroscience 166:157–167
9. Bolanos AR, Sarkisian M, Yang Y, Hori A, Helmers SL, Mikati M, Tandon P, Stafstrom CE, Holmes GL (1998) Comparison of valproate and phenobarbital treatment after status epilepticus in rats. Neurology 51(1):41–48
10. Bona E, Andersson AL, Blomgren K, Gilland E, Puka-Sundvall M, Gustafson K, Hagberg H (1999) Chemokine and inflammatory cell response to hypoxia-ischemia in immature rats. Pediatr Res 45:500–509
11. Brewster A, Bender RA, Chen Y, Dube C, Eghbal-Ahmadi M, Baram TZ (2002) Developmental febrile seizures modulate hippocampal gene expression of hyperpolarization-activated channels in an isoform- and cell-specific manner. J Neurosci 22:4591–4599
12. Burtrum D, Silverstein FS (1994) Hypoxic-ischemic brain injury stimulates glial fibrillary acidic protein mRNA and protein expression in neonatal rats. Exp Neurol 126: 112–118
13. Cantagrel S, Gressens P, Bodard S, Suc AL, Laugier J, Guilloteau D, Chalon S (2001) mRNA D(2) dopaminergic receptor expression after hypoxia-ischemia in rat immature brain. Biol Neonate 80:68–73
14. Cataltepe O, Barron TF, Heitjan DF, Vannucci RC, Towfighi J (1995) Effect of hypoxia/ischemia on bicuculline-induced seizures in immature rats: behavioral and electrocortical phenomena. Epilepsia 36:396–403
15. Cavalheiro EA, Silva DF, Turski WA, Calderazzo-Filho LS, Bortolotto ZA, Turski L (1987) The susceptibility of rats to pilocarpine-induced seizures is age-dependent. Brain Res 465:43–58
16. Cha BH, Silveira DC, Liu X, Hu Y, Holmes GL (2002) Effect of topiramate following recurrent and prolonged seizures during early development. Epilepsy Res 51(3):217–232
17. Chen K, Neu A, Howard AL, Földy C, Echegoyen J, Hilgenberg L, Smith M, Mackie K, Soltesz I (2007) Prevention of plasticity of endocannabinoid signaling inhibits persistent limbic hyperexcitability caused by developmental seizures. J Neurosci 27(1):46–58
18. Chiba S (1985) Long-term effect of postnatal hypoxia on the seizure susceptibility in rats. Life Sci 37:1597–1604
19. Christensen J, Pedersen MG, Pedersen CB, Sidenius P, Olsen J, Vestergaard M (2009) Long-term risk of epilepsy after traumatic brain injury in children and young adults: a population-based cohort study. Lancet 373(9669):1105–1110

20. Chronopoulos A, Stafstrom C, Thurber S, Hyde P, Mikati M, Holmes GL (1993) Neuroprotective effect of felbamate after kainic acid-induced status epilepticus. Epilepsia 34(2):359–366
21. Cilio MR, Bolanos AR, Liu Z, Schmid R, Yang Y, Stafstrom CE, Mikati MA, Holmes GL (2001) Anticonvulsant action and long-term effects of gabapentin in the immature brain. Neuropharmacology 40(1):139–147
22. Comi AM, Weisz CJ, Highet BH, Johnston MV, Wilson MA (2004) A new model of stroke and ischemic seizures in the immature mouse. Pediatr Neurol 31:254–257
23. Cowell RM, Xu H, Parent JM, Silverstein FS (2006) Microglial expression of chemokine receptor CCR5 during rat forebrain development and after perinatal hypoxia-ischemia. J Neuroimmunol 173:155–165
24. D'Ambrosio R, Fairbanks JP, Fender JS, Born DE, Doyle DL, Miller JW (2004) Post-traumatic epilepsy following fluid percussion injury in the rat. Brain 127(Pt 2):304–314
25. D'Ambrosio R, Fender JS, Fairbanks JP, Simon EA, Born DE, Doyle DL, Miller JW (2005) Progression from frontal-parietal to mesial-temporal epilepsy after fluid percussion injury in the rat. Brain 128(Pt 1):174–188
26. Dennis G Jr, Sherman BT, Hosack DA, Yang J, Gao W, Lane HC, Lempicki RA (2003) DAVID: database for annotation, visualization, and integrated discovery. Genome Biol 4:P3
27. Doverhag C, Hedtjarn M, Poirier F, Mallard C, Hagberg H, Karlsson A, Savman K (2010) Galectin-3 contributes to neonatal hypoxic-ischemic brain injury. Neurobiol Dis 38:36–46
28. Dube C, Chen K, Eghbal-Ahmadi M, Brunson K, Soltesz I, Baram TZ (2000) Prolonged febrile seizures in the immature rat model enhance hippocampal excitability long term. Ann Neurol 47:336–344
29. Dubé C, Richichi C, Bender RA, Chung G, Litt B, Baram TZ (2006) Temporal lobe epilepsy after experimental prolonged febrile seizures: prospective analysis. Brain 129: 911–922
30. Dubé CM, Ravizza T, Hamamura M, Zha Q, Keebaugh A, Fok K, Andres AL, Nalcioglu O, Obenaus A, Vezzani A, Baram TZ (2010) Epileptogenesis provoked by prolonged experimental febrile seizures: mechanisms and biomarkers. J Neurosci 30:7484–7494
31. Dugich-Djordjevic MM, Tocco G, Willoughby DA, Najm I, Pasinetti G, Thompson RF, Baudry M, Lapchak PA, Hefti F (1992) BDNF mRNA expression in the developing rat brain following kainic acid-induced seizure activity. Neuron 8:1127–1138
32. Echegoyen J, Armstrong C, Morgan RJ, Soltesz I (2009) Single application of a CB1 receptor antagonist rapidly following head injury prevents long-term hyperexcitability in a rat model. Epilepsy Res 85(1):123–127
33. Filloux FM, Adair J, Narang N (1996) The temporal evolution of striatal dopamine receptor binding and mRNA expression following hypoxia-ischemia in the neonatal rat. Brain Res Dev Brain Res 94:81–91
34. Friedman LK, Sperber EF, Moshe SL, Bennett MV, Zukin RS (1997) Developmental regulation of glutamate and GABA(A) receptor gene expression in rat hippocampus following kainate-induced status epilepticus. Dev Neurosci 19:529–542
35. Forsgren L, Beghi E, Oun A, Sillanpää M (2005) The epidemiology of epilepsy in Europe – a systematic review. Eur J Neurol 12(4):245–253
36. Galanopoulou AS, Buckmaster PS, Staley KJ, Moshé SL, Perucca E, Engel J Jr, Löscher W, Noebels JL, Pitkänen A, Stables J, White HS, O'Brien TJ, Simonato M, American Epilepsy Society Basic Science Committee And The International League Against Epilepsy Working Group On Recommendations For Preclinical Epilepsy Drug Discovery (2012) Identification of new epilepsy treatments: issues in preclinical methodology. Epilepsia 53(3):571–582
37. Gubits RM, Burke RE, Casey-McIntosh G, Bandele A, Munell F (1993) Immediate early gene induction after neonatal hypoxia-ischemia. Brain Res Mol Brain Res 18:228–238
38. Gulec G, Noyan B (2001) Do recurrent febrile convulsions decrease the threshold for pilocarpine-induced seizures? Effects of nitric oxide. Brain Res Dev Brain Res 126:223–228
39. Gurkoff GG, Giza CC, Hovda DA (2006) Lateral fluid percussion injury in the developing rat causes an acute, mild behavioral dysfunction in the absence of significant cell death. Brain Res 1077(1):24–36

40. Hagberg H, Gilland E, Bona E, Hanson LA, Hahin-Zoric M, Blennow M, Holst M, McRae A, Soder O (1996) Enhanced expression of interleukin (IL)-1 and IL-6 messenger RNA and bioactive protein after hypoxia-ischemia in neonatal rats. Pediatr Res 40:603–609
41. Hanaya R, Boehm N, Nehlig A (2007) Dissociation of the immunoreactivity of synaptophysin and GAP-43 during the acute and latent phases of the lithium-pilocarpine model in the immature and adult rat. Exp Neurol 204:720–732
42. Hedtjarn M, Mallard C, Eklind S, Gustafson-Brywe K, Hagberg H (2004) Global gene expression in the immature brain after hypoxia-ischemia. J Cereb Blood Flow Metab 24:1317–1332
43. Hedtjarn M, Mallard C, Hagberg H (2004) Inflammatory gene profiling in the developing mouse brain after hypoxia-ischemia. J Cereb Blood Flow Metab 24:1333–1351
44. Hirsch E, Baram TZ, Snead OC 3rd (1992) Ontogenic study of lithium-pilocarpine-induced status epilepticus in rats. Brain Res 583:120–126
45. Holmes GL, Weber DA (1985) Effects of hypoxic-ischemic encephalopathies on kindling in the immature brain. Exp Neurol 90:194–203
46. Holmes GL, Thompson JL (1988) Effects of kainic acid on seizure susceptibility in the developing brain. Brain Res 467:51–59
47. da Huang W, Sherman B, Lempicki RA (2009) Systematic and integrative analysis of large gene lists using DAVID bioinformatics resources. Nat Protoc 4:44–57
48. Ivacko J, Szaflarski J, Malinak C, Flory C, Warren JS, Silverstein FS (1997) Hypoxic-ischemic injury induces monocyte chemoattractant protein-1 expression in neonatal rat brain. J Cereb Blood Flow Metab 17:759–770
49. Jensen FE, Applegate C, Burchfiel J, Lombroso CT (1991) Differential effects of perinatal hypoxia and anoxia on long term seizure susceptibility in the rat. Life Sci 49:399–407
50. Jensen FE, Applegate CD, Holtzman D, Belin TR, Burchfiel JL (1991) Epileptogenic effect of hypoxia in the immature rodent brain. Ann Neurol 29:629–637
51. Jensen FE, Holmes GL, Lombroso CT, Blume HK, Firkusny IR (1992) Age-dependent changes in long-term seizure susceptibility and behavior after hypoxia in rats. Epilepsia 33(6):971–980
52. Jensen FE, Wang C, Stafstrom CE, Liu Z, Geary C, Stevens MC (1998) Acute and chronic increases in excitability in rat hippocampal slices after perinatal hypoxia in vivo. J Neurophysiol 79(1):73–81
53. Kadam SD, White AM, Staley KJ, Dudek FE (2010) Continuous electroencephalographic monitoring with radio-telemetry in a rat model of perinatal hypoxia-ischemia reveals progressive post-stroke epilepsy. J Neurosci 30:404–415
54. Kharatishvili I, Nissinen JP, McIntosh TK, Pitkänen A (2006) A model of posttraumatic epilepsy induced by lateral fluid-percussion brain injury in rats. Neuroscience 140(2):685–697
55. Klempt ND, Klempt M, Gunn AJ, Singh K, Gluckman PD (1992) Expression of insulin-like growth factor-binding protein 2 (IGF-BP 2) following transient hypoxia-ischemia in the infant rat brain. Brain Res Mol Brain Res 15:55–61
56. Kobayashi S, Welsh FA (1995) Regional alterations of ATP and heat-shock protein-72 mRNA following hypoxia-ischemia in neonatal rat brain. J Cereb Blood Flow Metab 15: 1047–1056
57. Koh S, Magid R, Chung H, Stine CD, Wilson DN (2007) Depressive behavior and selective downregulation of serotonin receptor expression after early-life seizures: reversal by environmental enrichment. Epilepsy Behav 10:26–31
58. Kornblum HI, Sankar R, Shin DH, Wasterlain CG, Gall CM (1997) Induction of brain derived neurotrophic factor mRNA by seizures in neonatal and juvenile rat brain. Brain Res Mol Brain Res 44:219–228
59. Kotsopoulos IA, van Merode T, Kessels FG, de Krom MC, Knottnerus JA (2002) Systematic review and meta-analysis of incidence studies of epilepsy and unprovoked seizures. Epilepsia 43(11):1402–1409
60. Kremlev SG, Roberts RL, Palmer C (2007) Minocycline modulates chemokine receptors but not interleukin-10 mRNA expression in hypoxic-ischemic neonatal rat brain. J Neurosci Res 85:2450–2459

61. Kubová H, Mareš P, Suchomelová L, Brožek G, Druga R, Pitkänen A (2004) Status epilepticus in immature rats leads to behavioural and cognitive impairment and epileptogenesis. Eur J Neurosci 19:3255–3265
62. Kubová H, Mareš P (2007) Hypoxia-induced changes of seizure susceptibility in immature rats are modified by vigabatrin. Epileptic Disord 9(Suppl 1):S36–S43
63. Kubová H (2009) Pharmacology of seizure drugs. In: Schwartzkroin P (ed) Encyclopedia of basic epilepsy research, vol 2. Academic, Oxford, pp 780–786
64. Kumral A, Genc S, Ozer E, Yilmaz O, Gokmen N, Koroglu TF, Duman N, Genc K, Ozkan H (2006) Erythropoietin downregulates bax and DP5 proapoptotic gene expression in neonatal hypoxic-ischemic brain injury. Biol Neonate 89:205–210
65. Lauren HB, Lopez-Picon FR, Korpi ER, Holopainen IE (2005) Kainic acid-induced status epilepticus alters GABA receptor subunit mRNA and protein expression in the developing rat hippocampus. J Neurochem 94:1384–1394
66. Lauren HB, Lopez-Picon FR, Brandt AM, Rios-Rojas CJ, Holopainen IE (2010) Transcriptome analysis of the hippocampal CA1 pyramidal cell region after kainic acid-induced status epilepticus in juvenile rats. PLoS One 5:e10733
67. Lee CL, Frost JD Jr, Swann JW, Hrachovy RA (2008) A new animal model of infantile spasms with unprovoked persistent seizures. Epilepsia 49(2):298–307
68. Leibovici A, Rossignol C, Montrowl JA, Erickson JD, Varoqui H, Watanabe M, Chaudhry FA, Bredahl MK, Anderson KJ, Weiss MD (2007) The effects of hypoxia-ischemia on neutral amino acid transporters in the developing rat brain. Dev Neurosci 29:268–274
69. Leite JP, Babb TL, Pretorius JK, Kuhlman PA, Yeoman KM, Mathern GW (1996) Neuron loss, mossy fiber sprouting, and interictal spikes after intrahippocampal kainate in developing rats. Epilepsy Res 26:219–231
70. Lemos T, Cavalheiro EA (1995) Suppression of pilocarpine-induced status late development of epilepsy in rats. Exp Brain Res 102:423–428
71. Little E, Tocco G, Baudry M, Lee AS, Schreiber SS (1996) Induction of glucose-regulated protein (glucose-regulated protein 78/BiP and glucose-regulated protein 94) and heat shock protein 70 transcripts in the immature rat brain following status epilepticus. Neuroscience 75:209–219
72. Lowenstein DH, Bleck T, Macdonald RL (1999) It's time to revise the definition of status epilepticus. Epilepsia 40:123–124
73. Lukasiuk K, Dabrowski M, Adach A, Pitkanen A (2006) Epileptogenesis-related genes revisited. Prog Brain Res 158:223–241
74. Lynch M, Sayin U, Bownds J, Janumpalli S, Sutula T (2000) Long-term consequences of early postnatal seizures on hippocampal learning and plasticity. Eur J Neurosci 12:2252–2264
75. Mátéffyová A, Otáhal J, Tsenov G, Mareš P, Kubová H (2006) Intrahippocampal injection of endothelin-1 in immature rats results in neuronal death, development of epilepsy, and behavioral abnormalities later in life. Eur J Neurosci 24:351–360
76. Matsumoto M (1990) The effects of perinatal hypoxia on pentylenetetrazol-induced seizures in developing rats. Life Sci 46:1787–1792
77. Menon DK, Schwab K, Wright DW, Maas AI, Demographics and Clinical Assessment Working Group of the International and Interagency Initiative toward Common Data Elements for Research on Traumatic Brain Injury and Psychological Health (2010) Position statement: definition of traumatic brain injury. Arch Phys Med Rehabil 91(11):1637–1640
78. Mikati MA, Holmes GL, Chronopoulos A, Hyde P, Thurber S, Gatt A, Liu Z, Werner S, Stafstrom CE (1994) Phenobarbital modifies seizure-related brain injury in the developing brain. Ann Neurol 36(3):425–433
79. Morioka I, Tsuneishi S, Takada S, Matsuo M (2004) PDGF-alpha receptor expression following hypoxic-ischemic injury in the neonatal rat brain. Kobe J Med Sci 50:21–30
80. Moshé SL, Albala BJ (1985) Perinatal hypoxia and subsequent development of seizures. Physiol Behav 35:819–823
81. Munell F, Burke RE, Bandele A, Gubits RM (1994) Localization of c-fos, c-jun, and hsp70 mRNA expression in brain after neonatal hypoxia-ischemia. Brain Res Dev Brain Res 77:111–121

82. Nehlig A, Motte J, Moshé SL, Plouin P (eds) (1999) Childhood epilepsies and brain development. John Libbey & Co, London, p 311
83. Nehlig A, Rudolf G, Leroy C, Rigoulot MA, Simpson IA, Vannucci SJ (2006) Pentylenetetrazol-induced status epilepticus up-regulates the expression of glucose transporter mRNAs but not proteins in the immature rat brain. Brain Res 1082:32–42
84. Neligan A, Shorvon SD (2011) Prognostic factors, morbidity and mortality in tonic-clonic status epilepticus: a review. Epilepsy Res 93(1):1–10
85. Ohno M, Sasahara M, Narumiya S, Tanaka N, Yamano T, Shimada M, Hazama F (1999) Expression of platelet-derived growth factor B-chain and beta-receptor in hypoxic/ischemic encephalopathy of neonatal rats. Neuroscience 90:643–651
86. Pitkänen A (2010) Therapeutic approaches to epileptogenesis–hope on the horizon. Epilepsia 51(Suppl 3):2–17
87. Pitkanen A, Lukasiuk K (2009) Molecular and cellular basis of epileptogenesis in symptomatic epilepsy. Epilepsy Behav 14(Suppl 1):16–25
88. Pitkanen A, Lukasiuk K (2011) Mechanisms of epileptogenesis and potential treatment targets. Lancet Neurol 10:173–186
89. Pitkänen A, Sutula TP (2002) Is epilepsy a progressive disorder? Prospects for new therapeutic approaches in temporal-lobe epilepsy. Lancet Neurol 1(3):173–181
90. Priel MR, dos Santos NF, Cavalheiro EA (1996) Developmental aspects of the pilocarpine model of epilepsy. Epilepsy Res 26:115–121
91. Porter BE, Cui XN, Brooks-Kayal AR (2006) Status epilepticus differentially alters AMPA and kainate receptor subunit expression in mature and immature dentate granule neurons. Eur J Neurosci 23:2857–2863
92. Rakhade SN, Klein PM, Huynh T, Hilario-Gomez C, Kosaras B, Rotenberg A, Jensen FE (2011) Development of later life spontaneous seizures in a rodent model of hypoxia-induced neonatal seizures. Epilepsia 52:753–765
93. Rizzi M, Perego C, Aliprandi M, Richichi C, Ravizza T, Colella D, Veliskova J, Moshe SL, De Simoni MG, Vezzani A (2003) Glia activation and cytokine increase in rat hippocampus by kainic acid-induced status epilepticus during postnatal development. Neurobiol Dis 14:494–503
94. Romijn HJ, Voskuyl RA, Coenen AM (1994) Hypoxic-ischemic encephalopathy sustained in early postnatal life may result in permanent epileptic activity and an altered cortical convulsive threshold in rat. Epilepsy Res 17:31–42
95. Sanchez RM, Jensen FE (2001) Maturational aspects of epilepsy mechanisms and consequences for the immature brain. Epilepsia 42:577–585
96. Sanchez RM, Koh S, Rio C, Wang C, Lamperti ED, Sharma D, Corfas G, Jensen FE (2001) Decreased glutamate receptor 2 expression and enhanced epileptogenesis in immature rat hippocampus after perinatal hypoxia-induced seizures. J Neurosci 21:8154–8163
97. Sankar R, Shin DH, Liu H, Mazarati A, Pereira de Vasconcelos A, Wasterlain CG (1998) Patterns of status epilepticus-induced neuronal injury during development and long-term consequences. J Neurosci 18:8382–8393
98. Sankar R, Shin D, Mazarati AM, Liu H, Katsumori H, Lezama R, Wasterlain CG (2000) Epileptogenesis after status epilepticus reflects age- and model-dependent plasticity. Ann Neurol 48:580–589
99. Santos NF, Marques RH, Correia L, Sinigaglia-Coimbra R, Calderazzo L, Sanabria ER, Cavalheiro EA (2000) Multiple pilocarpine-induced status epilepticus in developing rats: a long-term behavioral and electrophysiological study. Epilepsia 41(Suppl 6):S57–S63
100. Scantlebury MH, Gibbs SA, Foadjo B, Lema P, Psarropoulou C, Carmant L (2005) Febrile seizures in the predisposed brain: a new model of temporal lobe epilepsy. Ann Neurol 58:41–49
101. Scantlebury MH, Heida JG, Hasson HJ, Velísková J, Velísek L, Galanopoulou AS, Moshé SL (2007) Age-dependent consequences of status epilepticus: animal models. Epilepsia 48(Suppl 2):75–82
102. Scantlebury MH, Galanopoulou AS, Chudomelova L, Raffo E, Betancourth D, Moshé SL (2010) A model of symptomatic infantile spasms syndrome. Neurobiol Dis 37:604–612

103. Scott RC, Kirkham FJ (2007) Clinical update: childhood convulsive status epilepticus. Lancet 370(9589):724–726
104. Shimizu-Okabe C, Okabe A, Kilb W, Sato K, Luhmann HJ, Fukuda A (2007) Changes in the expression of cation-Cl- cotransporters, NKCC1 and KCC2, during cortical malformation induced by neonatal freeze-lesion. Neurosci Res 59:288–295
105. Spandou E, Papoutsopoulou S, Soubasi V, Karkavelas G, Simeonidou C, Kremenopoulos G, Guiba-Tziampiri O (2004) Hypoxia-ischemia affects erythropoietin and erythropoietin receptor expression pattern in the neonatal rat brain. Brain Res 1021:167–172
106. Stafstrom CE, Thompson JL, Holmes GL (1992) Kainic acid seizures in the developing brain: status epilepticus and spontaneous recurrent seizures. Brain Res Dev Brain Res 65:227–236
107. Stafström CE, Moshé SL, Swann JW, Nehlig A, Jacobs MP, Schwartzkroin PA (2006) Models of pediatric epilepsies: strategies and opportunities. Epilepsia 47:1407–1414
108. Statler KD, Swank S, Abildskov T, Bigler ED, White HS (2008) Traumatic brain injury during development reduces minimal clonic seizure thresholds at maturity. Epilepsy Res 80(2–3):163–170
109. Statler KD, Scheerlinck P, Pouliot W, Hamilton M, White HS, Dudek FE (2009) A potential model of pediatric posttraumatic epilepsy. Epilepsy Res 86(2–3):221–223
110. Suchomelová L, Baldwin R, Wasterlain CG (2006) The role of hyperthermia in status epilepticus-induced epileptogenesis. In: 60th AES annual meeting of the American Epilepsy Society, San Diego, 2006, Epilepsia 47, Suppl 4, Abst. (4.096)
111. Suchomelova L, Baldwin RA, Kubova H, Thompson KW, Sankar R, Wasterlain CG (2006) Treatment of experimental status epilepticus in immature rats: dissociation between anticonvulsant and antiepileptogenic effects. Pediatr Res 59(2):237–243
112. Tan Z, Sankar R, Shin D, Sun N, Liu H, Wasterlain CG, Schreiber SS (2002) Differential induction of p53 in immature and adult rat brain following lithium-pilocarpine status epilepticus. Brain Res 928:187–193
113. Theodore WH, Bhatia S, Hatta J, Fazilat S, DeCarli C, Bookheimer SY, Gaillard WD (1999) Hippocampal atrophy, epilepsy duration, and febrile seizures in patients with partial seizures. Neurology 52:132–136
114. Tsenov G, Mátéffyová A, Mareš P, Otáhal J, Kubová H (2007) Intrahippocampal injection of endothelin-1, a new model of ischemia-induced seizures in immature rats. Epilepsia 48(Suppl 5):7–13
115. Tsenov G, Kubová H, Mareš P (2008) Changes of cortical epileptic afterdischarges after status epilepticus in immature rats. Epilepsy Res 78:178–185
116. Velíšková J, Pitkanen A, Swartzkroin PA, Moshe SL (2006) Behavioral characterization of seizures in rats. In: Models of seizures and epilepsy. Elsevier, Amsterodam, pp 601–611
117. Walton M, Young D, Sirimanne E, Dodd J, Christie D, Williams C, Gluckman P, Dragunow M (1996) Induction of clusterin in the immature brain following a hypoxic-ischemic injury. Brain Res Mol Brain Res 39:137–152
118. Wang H, Yao Y, Jiang X, Chen D, Xiong Y, Mu D (2006) Expression of Nogo-A and NgR in the developing rat brain after hypoxia-ischemia. Brain Res 1114:212–220
119. Wang LY, Cai WQ, Chen PH, Deng QY, Zhao CM (2009) Downregulation of P2X7 receptor expression in rat oligodendrocyte precursor cells after hypoxia ischemia. Glia 57:307–319
120. Williams PA, Dou P, Dudek FE (2004) Epilepsy and synaptic reorganization in a perinatal rat model of hypoxia-ischemia. Epilepsia 45:1210–1218
121. Wilson DN, Chung H, Elliott RC, Bremer E, George D, Koh S (2005) Microarray analysis of postictal transcriptional regulation of neuropeptides. J Mol Neurosci 25:285–298
122. Yang JS, Yong DP, Hartlage PL (1995) Seizures associated with stroke in childhood. Pediatr Neurol 12:136–138
123. Zhang G, Raol YH, Hsu FC, Coulter DA, Brooks-Kayal AR (2004) Effects of status epilepticus on hippocampal GABAA receptors are age-dependent. Neuroscience 125:299–303
124. Zhao DY, Wu XR, Pei YQ, Zuo QH (1985) Long-term effects of febrile convulsion on seizure susceptibility in P77PMC rat–resistant to acoustic stimuli but susceptible to kainate-induced seizures. Exp Neurol 88:688–695

Paediatric Intractable Epilepsy Syndromes: Changing Concepts in Diagnosis and Management

Pamela L. Follett, Nitishkumar Vora, and J. Helen Cross

Contents

Abstract Epilepsy surgery for drug-resistant childhood epilepsy is not new. However, brain imaging, surgical and anaesthetic techniques have improved to the extent that they are now as much safer and realistic option than they were in the past. Further, the range of surgical candidates is wide, and previous concepts about likely surgical candidates are now challenged as children with previously thought widespread or apparent multifocal disease are evaluated. Outcomes for seizure freedom range from 40 to 80 % depending on the underlying aetiology and the extent of

P.L. Follett
Child Neurology, Lewis Rhodes Labs, Inc., Acton, MA, USA

N. Vora
Neurosciences Unit, Great Ormond Street Hospital for Children, London, UK

J.H. Cross (✉)
Neurosciences Unit, UCL-Institute of Child Health,
4/5 Long Yard, London WC1N 3LU, UK

Great Ormond Street Hospital for Children, London, UK

Young Epilepsy, Lingfield, UK
e-mail: h.cross@ucl.ac.uk

N. Akalan, C. Di Rocco (eds.), *Pediatric Epilepsy Surgery*,
Advances and Technical Standards in Neurosurgery,
DOI 10.1007/978-3-7091-1360-8_2, © Springer-Verlag Wien 2012

resection. However, the aims of surgery may include seizure reduction in some and improvement in neurodevelopment and behaviour in others, which are less predictable. Epilepsy surgery in children is no longer a last resort. Children thought to be likely candidates should be evaluated early in their natural history to optimise outcomes in the long term.

Keywords Epilepsy surgery • Childhood • MRI • Seizure outcome

Introduction

*Epilepsy i*s a chronic neurological condition characterised by recurrent epileptic seizures where an *epileptic seizure* can be defined as a transient occurrence of signs and/or symptoms due to abnormal, excessive or synchronous neuronal activity in the brain [20]. Five percent of the population will have a seizure during their lifetime. About 50 million people worldwide have epilepsy, and nearly two out of every three new cases are discovered in developing countries. Epilepsy is about twice as common in children as in adults, with a rate of 7/1,000 in childhood and only 3.3/1,000 in adults.

Anti-epileptic drugs (AEDs) are the first-line treatment, and seizures will be well controlled by medications in approximately two out of three children with epilepsy. Unfortunately, up to one third of children will not respond optimally to medical treatment, with either continued seizures or unacceptable side effects. Furthermore, there is a high rate of cognitive and behavioural disorders associated with early onset epilepsy. A proportion of these children may be candidates for *epilepsy surgery*, the removal or modification of part of the brain with the specific aim of treating epilepsy. This is not a new concept; it has been used in the management of epilepsy for over 100 years. However, it is only relatively recently that surgery has gained momentum as a realistic choice in the management of epilepsy in children.

The epidemiology of epilepsy differs between adults and children. Intractable epilepsy in adults is frequently caused by temporal lobe epilepsy (TLE). Temporal lobe resection for the treatment of TLE has provided an excellent option for patients. Excision of the seizure focus generates high expectations for seizure control, minimal loss of function and low morbidity [14, 44]. However, TLE is not a particularly common disorder in children. The underlying pathologies of paediatric epilepsy tend instead to involve extratemporal regions and present in a more diffuse manner. Furthermore, early life seizures more commonly arise secondary to a developmental disorder. These epilepsies can be catastrophic in onset, with developmental regression and related concerns that play a significant role in decision making [2]. This combination of factors results in a group of patients presenting with surgically remediable epilepsy in childhood who exhibit distinctly different characteristics from the typical adult presentation.

Many advances have occurred over the past 25 years since the early reports of successful epilepsy surgery in a highly selected paediatric population. There are increasing data on the benefit of epilepsy surgery in a wider range of carefully evaluated children [1, 27]. Improvements in seizure frequency and management are well documented, but consistent evidence of definable social and cognitive progress in this population has been elusive. A better understanding of the scope of positive and negative outcomes is essential. Expectations of benefit play a critical role in the decision-making process of not only on whom to operate but also when. Fortunately, numerous advances in presurgical evaluation, surgical methods and monitoring technology have improved decision making, procedural options and outcomes.

Evolving Methods and Perspectives

Candidate Selection: Expanding Criteria

Since the late nineteenth century, surgery has been utilised as a treatment for medically refractory epilepsy and recognised as possibly relevant in children over the past 50 years. Depending on the specific procedure, current chances of seizure remission following resective surgery of the epileptogenic focus in adults are typically in the range of 60–70 % [14] and the risk of complications and associated morbidity remains low. Many referrals for epilepsy surgery in the paediatric population are for catastrophic onset epilepsies. Initial reluctance to consider children as candidates for epilepsy surgery has been shown to be unfounded [10]. Success rates in children also vary with the specific procedure and the causative pathology but can be impressive, with low morbidity and mortality rates when candidates are evaluated and treated in specialist paediatric centres. It is currently estimated that 127 children in every 1,000,000 present with drug-resistant epilepsy each year, of which one in five will be appropriate candidates for a surgical procedure [5].

Surgery is considered for drug-resistant epilepsy in children when an assessment indicates that there will be a significant improvement in seizure control in the absence of an unacceptable loss of function. Meeting the first requirement of these criteria would appear straightforward; drug-resistant epilepsy is that which does not respond to medical intervention. Nonetheless, adult definitions have not necessarily been relevant to the childhood population. Over time it has become evident that the traditional view of *drug resistance* – failure of two drugs over 2 years – is not applicable in many, particularly those with seizure onset within the first 2 years of life [4]. More recently, the ILAE has put forward a modified definition of *treatment failure:* 'adequate trials of two tolerated and appropriately chosen AED schedules (whether as monotherapies or in combination) that fail to achieve sustained seizure freedom'. In this report, treatment response is defined as seizure freedom lasting at least three times the longest seizure-free interval prior to a new intervention [33]. This would take into consideration even the very young with more catastrophic onset epilepsy.

Additional uncertainty surrounds the developmental delay, cognitive decline and social costs associated with unremitting seizures in children [11]. Considerable concern that developmental losses may become less remediable over time adds a sense of potential urgency to the decision [16, 17]. This is further exacerbated by the catastrophic nature of seizures in some young children.

Historically, impaired intellectual function has been interpreted to mean widespread brain disorder predictive of a poor surgical outcome. Consistent with this belief, criteria for consideration of epilepsy surgery have included normal IQ in some circumstances [38]. However, outcome studies in children suggest that impaired IQ is not synonymous with poor seizure outcome. If a child's cognitive disabilities are at least in part a consequence of ongoing seizures, there is additional potential for improvement in their achievements following surgery with seizure control. There are also a number of studies that have shown significant gains in IQ testing over time after attaining seizure-free status with epilepsy surgery [2, 21, 45]. These children present a compelling argument for a greater sense of urgency to proceed with epilepsy surgery.

Children with epilepsy frequently have coexistent psychiatric disorders. More than half of children with both seizures and a structural brain abnormality will have a psychiatric disorder. Thus the rate of psychiatric disorder in children coming in for surgical evaluation is particularly high. This has been demonstrated in children with either extratemporal [9] or temporal lobe epilepsy [37]. Unfortunately, the group of children with relevant cognitive and behavioural comorbidities may not experience significant improvement in these disabilities following epilepsy surgery [21, 37]; some diagnoses may indeed evolve. Although some children gain additional psychiatric diagnoses following epilepsy surgery despite an improvement in seizure control, there is no indication that the surgery increases this risk. Appropriate counselling of families is essential prior to surgery in order to highlight this but it is evident that existing psychiatric disorders do not represent a contraindication to surgery.

Surgical Techniques for Childhood Epilepsies

Surgery is considered for drug-resistant epilepsy when an assessment indicates the potential for significant improvement in seizure control in the absence of an unacceptable loss of function. Outcomes are optimal when seizures are demonstrated to arise from one well-defined area that can be removed without functional compromise. This was initially restricted to a temporal lobectomy procedure performed in adults; however, studies showed that many of the adults who benefitted from this intervention had epilepsy since early childhood, suggesting the potential for similar surgery in children [51].

At this time it is well recognised that the complete resection of a single discrete seizure focus in a non-eloquent region of cortex provides an excellent option for seizure treatment at any age. However, the increasing scope of paediatric patients presenting for surgery includes children with syndromes where seizures may be perceived to be generalised or multifocal in onset. Both the site of onset and pathogenesis differentiate paediatric from adult epilepsy [26] (Tables 1 and 2). Advances

Table 1 Distribution of procedures undertaken in children undergoing epilepsy surgery from a survey undertaken in 2004 ($N=543$) [26]

Procedure	% (N)
Resections/diagnostic electrodes	81 (440)
Hemispherectomy	15.8 (86)
Multilobar	12.9 (86)
Lobar/focal	48 (261)
Temporal	23.2 (126)
Frontal	17.5 (95)
Parietal	2.8 (15)
Occipital	1.7 (9)
Diagnostic electrodes only	3.7 (20)
Multiple sub-pial transection	0.6 (3)
Vagal nerve stimulator	15.8 (86)
Corpus callosotomy	3.1 (17)

Table 2 Underlying pathologies in children undergoing surgery for epilepsy [26]

Pathology	% (N)
Cortical dysplasia	42.4 (175)
Tumour	19.1 (79)
Atrophy/stroke	9.9 (41)
Hippocampal sclerosis	6.5 (27)
Gliosis/normal pathology	6.3 (26)
Tuberous sclerosis complex	5.1 (21)
Hypothalamic hamartoma	3.6 (15)
Sturge Weber syndrome	2.9 (12)
Rasmussen syndrome	2.7 (11)
Vascular (not Sturge Weber)	1.5 (6)

in neuroimaging and neuroanaesthesia have reduced the morbidity and further widened the spectrum of surgical candidates. Improved MRI techniques for structural imaging, as well as more options for functional assessment, have informed preoperative analysis. Advances in surgery such as image-guided techniques, prolonged video EEG and invasive monitoring with stimulation for eloquent cortex have significantly improved surgery outcomes [12]. These techniques can facilitate the goal of complete removal of a seizure focus with preservation of function and fewer complications for a greater range of patients.

Surgical options are considered in two categories: resective and functional. Hemispherectomy and multilobar procedures are the procedures most commonly undertaken in children, especially in the very young [18, 26]. Extratemporal resection for focal cortical dysplasia and developmental tumours is more common in older children with good results [1, 19, 27, 29].

The most common causes of drug-resistant seizures in children are cortical malformations [24]. A number are too diffuse to be addressed with a single resective procedure. However, when restricted to a single hemisphere, variable degrees of resection have been shown to be successful. Although large areas of malformation may be easily recognised (Fig. 1), others are more subtle but the introduction and utilisation of higher resolution MR imaging has made it increasingly clear that cortical dysplasia is an

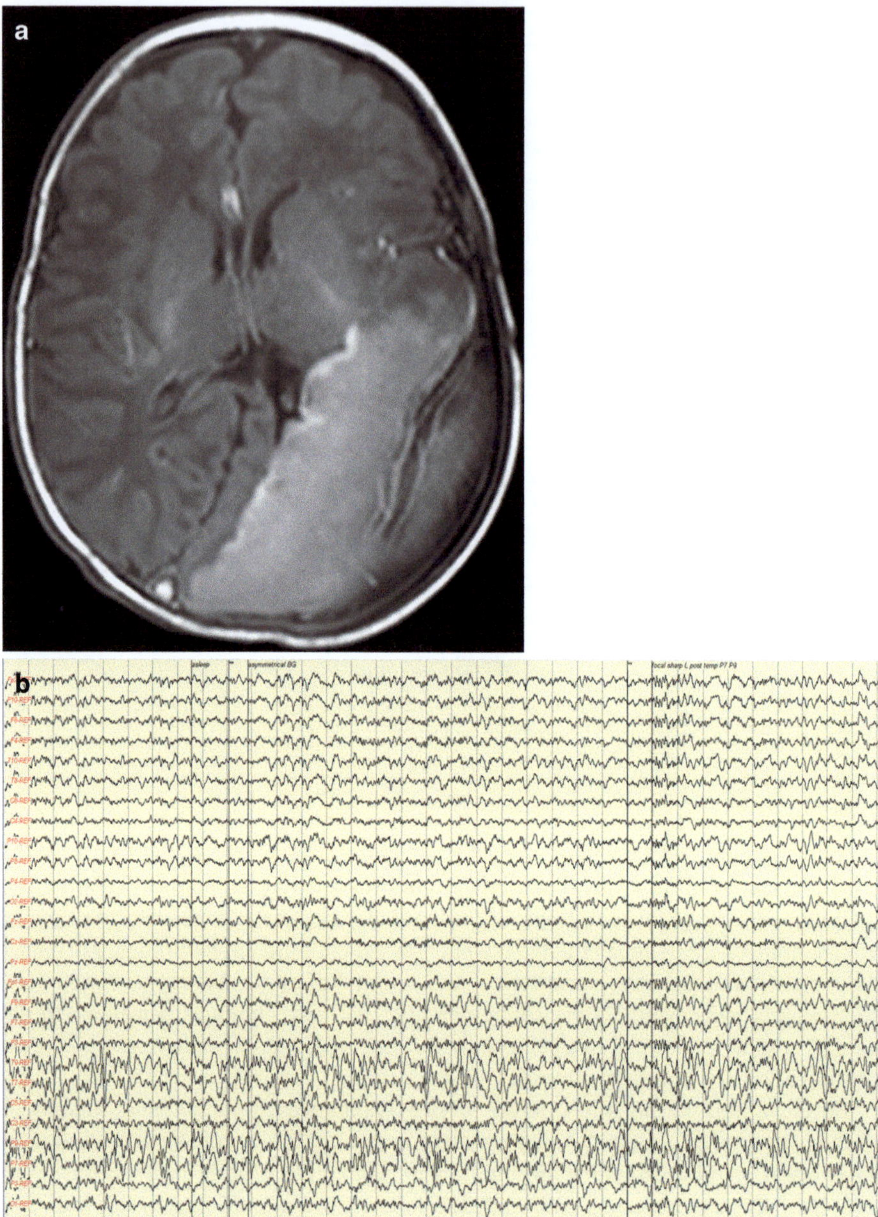

Fig. 1 MRI (**a**) and EEG (**b**) of an infant presenting with seizures in the neonatal period. The MRI shows left hemimegalancephaly; the EEG seizure onset in the left hemisphere. The child underwent a left functional hemispherectomy at 4 months of age, leading to seizure freedom

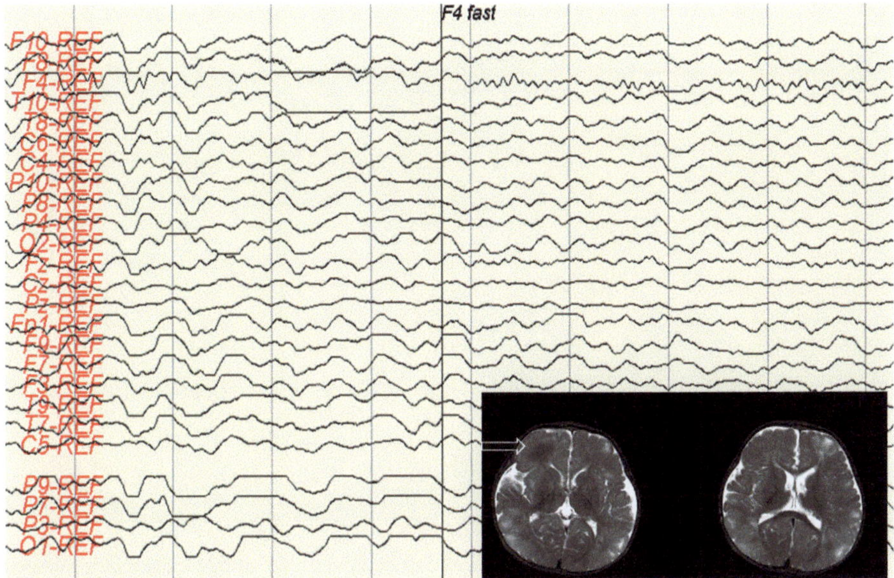

Fig. 2 MRI and ictal EEG of a 15-month old with focal seizures, the result of tuberous sclerosis. Ictal EEG showed seizure onset from the right frontal region (F4). Although there are multiple tubers seen on MRI, there is a large calcified tuber in the left frontal region (*arrowed*). Removal of the right frontal tuber led to seizure freedom for 3 years

extremely common cause of childhood epilepsy. When these lesions can be identified and are not in eloquent cortex, surgical excision is a highly effective option. Unfortunately, these lesions are found at a surprisingly high frequency in areas of critical, functional cortex. Thus a complete evaluation of both the structure and functionality of the region of interest is essential before surgery can be considered [26, 34].

The types of seizures seen in the early onset epilepsies are more a reflection of the age of presentation than the underlying pathology. For example, infantile spasms are events that occur in infants as an age-specific response to a range of pathologies involving a single discrete malformation, multiple foci or a diffuse area of the brain. Thus an apparent generalised event can reflect the immaturity of the environment as opposed to indicating pathology. In cases where the underlying pathology is discrete and identifiable, prompt surgery may provide the best treatment option. The developmental regression that occurs in the presence of unremitting seizures is typically devastating, and earlier surgery is associated with better postsurgical developmental outcomes [28]. In addition, the very young brain retains the ability to alter its functional architecture in response to surgical excision and thus preservation of eloquent cortex is less of a concern.

Early onset epilepsy, especially those related to particular pathologies such as Sturge-Weber syndrome, tuberous sclerosis (Fig. 2), hemispheric syndromes and

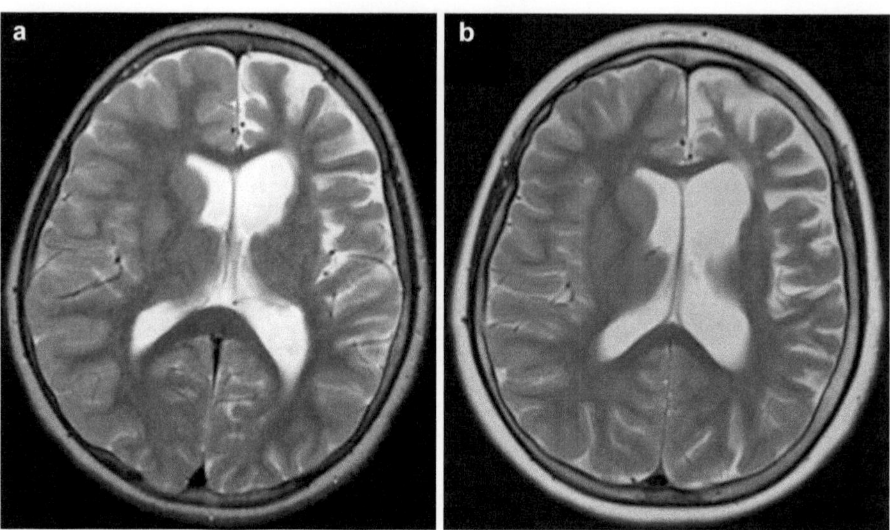

Fig. 3 Sequential MRI of the brain of an 8 year old who presented with R focal motor seizures, and subsequently developed increasing frequency to Epilepsia partialis continua with increasing right hemiparesis. Although atrophy of the left hemisphere is seen on the first scan (**a**), this has progressed on the second scan 12 months later (**b**) suggestive of Rasmussen encephalitis

extensive focal cortical dysplasia, can present with generalised or multifocal features both in clinical presentation and EEG characteristics. However, with underlying focal/lateralised pathology, they are likely to have focal onset and can break traditional concepts of epilepsy surgery [28]. Further with more advanced analysis of epileptic activity, increasingly complex excisions are being evaluated for TS that can be highly successful [49].

A procedure considered far more frequently in children than in adults is hemispheric disconnection. This is due in part to the spectrum of underlying pathology as well as to the catastrophic and progressive nature of these diagnoses. For example, seizures are common in Sturge-Weber syndrome, a sporadically occurring disorder with leptomeningeal angioma and associated facial capillary haemangioma (port-wine stain). Seizures can be difficult to control especially if they commence before 1 year as they do in over half of the children. When the seizures do not respond to medical treatment and the process is hemispheric and unilateral, then a hemispherectomy can be a highly beneficial intervention. These children typically present with a hemiparesis that may progress with seizures. Timing of surgery is an issue as some studies indicate a better outcome with early resective surgery [8, 32]. The several different types of hemispherectomy procedures considered under these circumstances have been shown to have similar outcomes [27].

Another paediatric disorder treated with hemispherectomy is Rasmussen Encephalitis (RE). RE is a rare presumed autoimmune disorder involving unilateral hemispheric inflammation and in many relentless epileptic encephalopathy (Fig. 3). Seizures are frequently intractable and progression of the disease leads to cortical hemiatrophy and contralateral hemiparesis. Hemispherectomy is the only cure. It improves epilepsy and halts the cognitive regression, but results in a dense hemiparesis and hemianopia. The most challenging aspect of the treatment debate involves the timing of surgery, as outcomes are reported as better with earlier intervention but not all children may progress to the level of disability achieved by surgery [6]. Hemispherectomies are also considered in children with extensive malformations when the pathology appears to be limited to one side of the brain.

Options are more limited when a seizure focus cannot be identified or when a recognised focus is inextricably linked with essential eloquent cortex. When the child's epilepsy is intractable and debilitating but the cause is not amenable to resection, functional surgical interventions may be considered. The intent of these procedures is to disrupt seizure propagation and contain the abnormal activity as much as possible. Corpus callosotomy, the severing of the connecting fibres between the two hemispheres of the brain, is one such procedure. The goal is to restrict epileptic activity to one hemisphere. This procedure has provided significant relief for 'drop' attacks that cause injury, markedly improving quality of life [36, 41]. Although drop attacks are the seizure type most consistently treated in this manner, improvement in other generalised seizures may also be experienced in individuals following surgery.

Multiple subpial transections is another palliative technique used where the surgical focus may be associated with functional cortex. The theory is that the process involves transection of the transverse fibres most implicated in seizure propagation while preserving the vertical functional pathways of the cortex. The technique has also been used in combination with respective surgery where the focus involves eloquent cortex [47] The technique has also been helpful in drug-resistant cases of Landau-Kleffner syndrome, an acquired epileptic aphasia associated with continuous spike-wave of slow sleep. In the absence of a discrete lesion, subpial transections are performed over Wernnicke's area (and deep into the sylvian fissure, under cortigographic guidance) on the EEG driving side in order to disrupt the epileptic focus while retaining relative preservation of the functional cortex [3, 39].

Timing of Surgery: The Role of Plasticity

The decision of the optimal timing of surgical treatment is often challenging, as the risk–benefit assessment requires clinical experience and multidisciplinary input. There are reasons specific to early life brain development why surgery should be considered promptly in the natural history of paediatric epilepsy. The first years of life are a critical period for the development of cognitive abilities. Studies demonstrate that the presence of seizures leads to cognitive impairment independently of underlying pathology [40]. When ongoing epileptic activity is at least in part responsible for cognitive dysfunction, improved outcome would be expected if and when seizure freedom can be achieved. Thus surgical intervention can be urgent in infants with catastrophic epilepsy unresponsive to medical intervention in order to try to prevent developmental regression or arrest. These candidates for epilepsy surgery need to be identified early in the process of the disease to prevent the possibility of worsening developmental outcomes that could be seen with delayed time to surgery.

There have been indications of ongoing reluctance to refer children for surgery. This barrier has resulted in many children experiencing an unnecessary wait for a possible curative procedure [26]. Epilepsy surgery in children under 3 years of age offers suitable candidates a good chance of significantly improved seizure outcome which compares with rates in older cohorts [16, 18] yet only a third of eligible children are referred within 2 years of diagnosis [26]. This is especially unfortunate since outcomes for cognitive testing, social determinants and motor recovery are all improved by earlier interventions that give the developing brain ample opportunity to develop compensatory function [12].

While the remarkable plasticity of the immature brain is a liability with progressive seizures, it is clearly an asset to epilepsy treatment outcomes. The child's brain is capable of significant reorganisation of neurological function after insult and surgery, highlighting the importance of early surgical intervention to prevent developmental arrest or regression [23]. Delay to surgery is associated with increased psychosocial, behavioural and educational problems. There are deficits not only associated with the presence of seizures but also with the existence of competitive, dysfunctional brain that can interfere with compensatory function in more functional brain regions [40]. Functional plasticity is particularly noted in the pattern of recovery of linguistic competence following dominant hemispherectomy in children with acquired epilepsy [7]. In congenital hemispheric disorders associated with epilepsy, the contralateral hemisphere is likely to develop dominance. When acquired disorders such as RE involve the dominant hemisphere, surgery at a younger age may provide a better opportunity for transfer of language function due to this increased plasticity. However, when disease progression is slow and deficits less profound, determining the optimum timing for surgery can be very challenging.

Another complication of the aspect of timing relates to the determinants of why children with epilepsy have such a high rate of cognitive disorders. There is evidence supporting hypotheses that seizures and altered cognition independently occur in the presence of the developmental brain pathologies that cause seizures. When the interaction between epilepsy and cognitive disability is uncertain, the necessity of surgery to prevent harm becomes less obvious [13].

Presurgical Evaluation

Management of epilepsy requires a multidisciplinary approach throughout the preoperative, perioperative and postoperative periods [12]. An appropriate team can properly address not only seizure management but also critical comorbidities such as safety, independence, mobility, emotional and behavioural issues, cognition, education and learning. The quality of life of patients and families is greatly enhanced by identifying and managing these additional risk factors.

Improved referral patterns are essential to optimising surgical outcomes [12]. Due to the need for appropriate technology, experience and expertise, children with drug-resistant epilepsy benefit when referred to comprehensive epilepsy centres rather than isolated surgical units. Children with behavioural or developmental regression in the setting of drug-resistant seizures should be referred with greater urgency for presurgical evaluation. Certain subgroups of surgical candidates should be referred to an experienced surgical unit equipped with multidisciplinary personnel with access to advanced technologies such as PET, SPECT and functional MRI. These subgroups would include particularly young children or those at greater risk for complications and morbidity, such as when a seizure focus is difficult to localise or in a potentially eloquent region where invasive EEG monitoring may be required.

Advances in structural imaging have led to improvements in identification of the areas responsible for seizure onset. As might be expected, surgical outcomes are improved when the pathological assessment of the resected region shows an abnormality [52]. Newer techniques in MRI imaging have improved the presurgical structural analysis such that the areas of abnormal cortex are more likely to be closely identified. 3D analysis, specific protocols of ultra-thin slices and additional types of echo sequences have greatly increased the sensitivity and specificity of MRI [22].

In order to optimise post-surgical outcome, it is not only critical to assess the brain being considered for resection, but also that the remaining brain is structurally normal. This is especially important when considering a wide resection or hemispherectomy, although subtle contralateral abnormalities may not be a contraindication to surgery [25]. Advances in functional imaging with fMRI have improved safety of resection by identifying areas of cortical function. When the presence of a structural lesion correlates with a specific electrographic seizure focus, the decision for surgical potential may be easy. In the absence of such helpful associations, non-invasive functional imaging may provide information about the likely area responsible. These studies can take the form of ictal and interictal single-photon emission computed tomography (SPECT) or interictal positron emission tomography (PET) [30].

At a minimum, surgical candidates should be evaluated with an interictal EEG that includes sleep monitoring, preferably video EEG monitoring, an MRI with a specified epilepsy protocol, and an age-appropriate neuropsychological and developmental assessment [12]. However, even with newer functional modalities invasive EEG monitoring may be necessary if a focus is particularly difficult to identify or if the interaction with eloquent cortex is indeterminate. Surgical decisions are mainly based on non-invasive monitoring with aid of functional imaging as needed. There is recognised need for invasive monitoring in selected cases, particularly when there is a delineated focus on EEG but MRI is either lesion-negative or the extent of the lesion cannot be defined. When more extensive assessment is indicated, then a child should be transferred to a specialist surgical centre with experience of such techniques.

Table 3 Engel classification system of postoperative outcomes

Class I – free of disabling seizures
Class II – rare disabling seizures
Class III – worthwhile improvement
Class IV – no worthwhile improvement

Outcomes

The primary objective of epilepsy surgery is seizure freedom, or at the very least reduction of seizures. It may also be aimed at improving other important aspects of neurodevelopment and quality of life. While complete resection of a seizure focus is the best predictor of seizure freedom, developmental outcomes have proven more difficult to quantify. Outcome goals need to be assessed with an individual focus, as population goals may be less appropriate to the spectrum of children appropriate for surgery. Now that low IQ, mental illness and very young age are not considered contraindications to a surgical approach, children being evaluated have an even greater range of developmental status specifically related to their underlying condition.

Nonetheless, relief from seizures remains the defined goal of epilepsy surgery. A number of classification schemes are used to assess outcome. The Engel classification system, originally devised in 1987, is the most commonly used scale (see Table 3) [50]. It identifies significant decreases in seizure number, but also allows for quantification of worthwhile improvement independent of decreased frequency. A change in severity of seizures, or decrease in a particularly troublesome seizure type such as drop attacks, can be reflected in this lifestyle-relevant category. This aside, categories are quite broad, and can be difficult to apply to some of the catastrophic onset epilepsies.

Epilepsy surgery is targeted towards seizure freedom or where possible, although in some with more complex epilepsy reduction in seizures may be the aim (Engel Grade I or II). Overall clinical outcomes appear to be dependent on several factors but the most important determinant of whether seizure freedom will be achieved postoperatively remains whether the resection of the seizure focus is complete [19, 34]. Currently, surgical outcome in children following focal resections is similar to that in adults, with seizure-free rates in the range of 75–80 %, particularly in patients with well-circumscribed lesions where complete lesion resection without sacrifice of functional brain is possible [46]. Children undergoing temporal lobe resection are more likely to achieve seizure freedom (85 %) [45] than those undergoing extratemporal resection (60 %) [29]. Seizure remission rates after surgery for extratemporal apparent non-lesional epilepsy are less favourable, typically due to the challenges of accomplishing a complete resection [34].

While all assessed groups demonstrate worthwhile levels of seizure reduction, cognitive, social and behavioural improvements remain more difficult to quantify. A reduction in the burden of ongoing epilepsy should confer psychosocial benefit and improve quality of life in children. Furthermore, surgical intervention at an earlier age could be expected to have a greater role in preventing cognitive dysfunction than would that in older patients. However, there are minimal published data to support these concepts. Accurate assessment of cognition, behaviour, psychosocial adaptation and quality of life are crucial for an understanding of paediatric epilepsy surgery candidates [12]. Children with ongoing seizures can experience a widening gap in IQ learning relative to their peers with consequent decrease in. Thus the maintenance of IQ in children following surgery could be interpreted as success.

Improvements in cognitive outcomes have been shown in early IQ/DQ in very young children after surgery. Younger children, the group that has highest deficits going into surgery, show the most benefit [35, 43]. Postoperative developmental trajectories are maintained with a stable velocity and importantly accelerated development may occur in seizure-free patients [21]. Furthermore, surgery for TLE performed in childhood results in additional long-term benefits in cognitive development with improved IQ seen beyond 6 years following surgery, related to seizure freedom and wean from medication [45].

The mechanisms underlying short-term and long-term cognitive advances may differ. Whereas short-term improvements may relate to the immediate cessation of seizure activity, long-term improvements have also been shown to be not only associated with seizure control but also removal of AEDs and increased grey matter volumes [45]. A wean from AEDs is a common goal following epilepsy surgery, particularly for parents who already perceive benefits of this objective. However, this may be yet another complex decision since recent tendencies towards less aggressive medication withdrawal are thought to be a contributing reason for improving outcomes following paediatric epilepsy surgery [27].

Patients with acquired disorders treated with a hemispherectomy consistently do better on follow up than children with congenital disorders, especially malformations. Postoperative seizure freedom in the group with developmental pathology is closer to 30 %, in contrast to those with acquired pathology who enjoy complete seizure remission over 80 % of the time [15]. Although most patients with more extensive surgery tend towards more moderate improvement, there are also gains in the social and cognitive outcomes of children after hemispherectomy. Immediate cognitive gains are reported in all groups following surgery, particularly in circumstances where the presence of seizures limits the child's exposure to social and environmental stimuli [48]. In studies with higher presurgical scores, there is less improvement in cognitive development; however, long-term outcomes are quite favourable in some groups [15, 42]. In patients treated with hemispherectomy for RE, language is significantly more impaired for left (presumed dominant) than right hemispherectomy and cognitive measures change little between surgery and follow up [42].

Significant behavioural improvements however are consistently appreciated post-hemispherectomy in children with unmanageable aggressive and explosive behaviours prior to surgery. This situation is most frequently noted in children with congenital hemiplegic syndromes the result of developmental pathologies whose postoperative seizure profile is the least encouraging of the groups [15]. This suggests that a realistic appraisal of prognosis requires an assessment of underlying pathology as patients with acquired or progressive disorders will have a differing prognosis than patients with congenital disorders both for seizure and behaviour outcome.

Conclusions

Advances in evaluation and surgery mean that wider spectrum of children are amenable to safe surgical resection. Not only can resective surgery for focal epilepsy in children result in similar levels of seizure remission to that seen in adults, surgery can provide a critical option to improve outcomes for a wide variety of paediatric epilepsies. Possible candidates can and should be identified early in their natural history and evaluated. All children with intractable epilepsy and evidence of a focal structural brain abnormality should be considered as possible candidates. This must actively include children under the age of 2 years, particularly those children with epilepsies that are likely to have a poor progress for seizure control. Furthermore, children with focal-onset epilepsy and a history of medication resistance should be considered even where a structural brain abnormality is not demonstrated, as further evaluation with advanced techniques may reveal that surgery is a possibility. Much can be gained from early referral when surgery may be deemed an appropriate option – much can be lost in the long term by delaying.

References

1. Ansari SF et al (2010) Surgery for extratemporal nonlesional epilepsy in children: a meta-analysis. Childs Nerv Syst 26(7):945–951
2. Battaglia D et al (2006) Cognitive assessment in epilepsy surgery of children. Childs Nerv Syst 22:744–759
3. Benifla M et al (2006) Multiple subpial transections in pediatric epilepsy: indications and outcomes. Childs Nerv Syst 22:992–998
4. Berg AT, Levy SR, Testa FM, D'Souza R (2009) Remission of epilepsy after 2 drug failures in children: a prospective study. Ann Neurol 65(5):510–519
5. Berg AT et al (2009) Frequency, prognosis and surgical treatment of structural abnormalities seen with magnetic resonance imaging in childhood epilepsy. Brain 132:2785–2797
6. Bien CG et al (2005) Pathogenesis, diagnosis and treatment of Rasmussen encephalitis: a European consensus statement. Brain 128:454–471
7. Boatman D et al (1999) Language recovery after left hemispherectomy in children with late-onset seizures. Ann Neurol 46(4):579–586
8. Bourgeois M et al (2007) Surgical treatment of epilepsy in Sturge-Weber syndrome in children. J Neurosurg 106(1):20–28
9. Colonnelli MC et al (2012) Psychopathology in children before and after surgery for extratemporal lobe epilepsy. Dev Med Child Neurol 54:521–526. doi:10.1111/j.1469-8749.2012.04293.x, first published on-line 14 Apr 2012
10. Cross JH (1999) Update on surgery for epilepsy. Arch Dis Child 81:356–359
11. Cross JH (2002) Epilepsy surgery in childhood. Epilepsia 43(S3):65–70
12. Cross JH et al (2006) Proposed criteria for referrral and evaluation of children for epilepsy surgery: recommendations of the subcommission for pediatric epilepsy surgery. Epilepsia 47(6):952–959
13. D'Argenzio L et al (2011) Cognitive outcome after extratemporal epilepsy surgery in childhood. Epilepsia 52(11):1966–1972
14. de Tisi J et al (2011) The long-term outcome of adult epilepsy surgery, patterns of seizure remission, and relapse: a cohort study. Lancet 378:1388–1395

15. Devlin AM et al (2003) Clinical outcomes of hemispherectomy for epilepsy in childhood and adolescence. Brain 126:556–566
16. Duchowny M et al (1998) Epilepsy surgery in the first three years of life. Epilepsia 39(7): 737–743
17. Dunkley C, Cross JH (2006) NICE guidelines and the epilepsies: How should practice change? Arch Dis Child 91:525–528
18. Dunkley C et al (2011) Epilepsy surgery in children under 3 years. Epilepsy Res 93:96–106
19. Edwards JC et al (2000) Seizure outcome after surgery for epilepsy due to malformaiton of cortical development. Neurology 55(8):1110–1114
20. Fisher RS et al (2005) Epileptic seizures and epilepsy: definitions proposed by the International League Against Epilepsy (ILAE) and the International Bureau for Epilpesy (IBE). Epilepsia 46(4):470–472
21. Freitag H, Tuxhorn I (2005) Cognitive function in preschool children after epilepsy surgery: rationale for early intervention. Epilepsia 46(4):561–567
22. Gaillard WD et al (2009) Guidelines for imaging infants and children with recent-onset epilepsy. Epilepsia 50(9):2147–2153
23. Gleissner U et al (2005) Greater functional recovery after temporal lobe epilepsy surgery in children. Brain 128:2822–2829
24. Guerrini R, Dobyns WB, Barkovitch AJ (2007) Abnormal development of the human cerebral cortex: genetics, functional consequences and treatment options. Trends Neurosci 31(3): 154–162
25. Hallbook T et al (2010) Contralateral MRI abnormalities in candidates for hemispherectomy for refractory epilepsy. Epilepsia 51(4):556–563
26. Harvey S, Cross JH, Shinnar S, Mathern BW (2008) Defining the spectrum of international practice in pediatric epilepsy surgery patients. Epilepsia 46(1):146–155
27. Hemb M et al (2010) Improved outcomes in pediatric epilepsy surgery: the UCLA experience. Neurology 74:1768–1775
28. Jonas R et al (2005) Surgery for symptomatic infant-onset epileptic encephalopathy with and without infantile spasms. Neurology 64:746–750
29. Kan P, Van Orman C, Kestle JRW (2008) Outcomes after surgery for focal epilepsy in children. Childs Nerv Syst 24:587–591
30. Knowlton RC et al (2008) Functional imaging: II. Prediction of epilepsy surgery outcome. Ann Neurol 64:35–41
31. Kossoff EH, Buck C, Freeman JM (2002) Outcomes of 32 hemispherectomies for Sturge-Weber sundrome worldwide. Neurology 59(11):1735–1738
32. Kramer U, Kahana E, Shorer Z, Ben-Zeev B (2000) Outcome of infants with unilateral Sturge-Weber syndrome and early onset seizures. Dev Med Child Neurol 42:756–759
33. Kwan P et al (2010) Definition of drug resistant epilepsy: consensus proposal by the ad hoc Task Force of the ILAE Commission on Therapeutic Strategies. Epilepsia 51(6):1069–1077
34. Lerner JT et al (2009) Assessment and surgical outcomes for mild type I and severe type II cortical dysplasia: a critical review and the UCLA experience. Epilepsia 50(6):1310–1335
35. Loddenkemper T et al (2007) Developmental outcome after epilepsy surgery in infancy. Pediatrics 119(5):930–935
36. Maehara T, Shimizu H (2001) Surgical outcome of corpus callosotomy in patients with drop attacks. Epilepsia 42(1):67–71
37. McLellan A et al (2005) Psychopathology in children with epilepsy before and after temporal lobe resection. Dev Med Child Neurol 47:666–672
38. Mohamed A et al (2001) Temporal lobe epilepsy due to hippocampal sclerosis in pediatric candidates for epilepsy surgery. Neurology 56(12):1643–1649
39. Morrell F et al (1995) Landau-Kleffner syndrome: treatment with subpial intracortical transection. Brain 118:1529–1546
40. Muter V, Taylor S, Vargha-Khadem F (1997) A longitudinal study of early intellectual development in hemiplegic children. Neuropsychologia 35(3):289–298

41. Nei M, O'Connor M, Liporace J, Sperling MR (2006) Refractory generalized seizures: response to corpus callosotomy and vagal nerve stimulation. Epilepsia 47(1):115–122
42. Pulsifer MB et al (2004) The cognitive outcome of hemispherectomy in 71 children. Epilepsia 45(3):243–254
43. Roulet-Perez E et al (2010) Impact of severe epilepsy on development: recovery potential after successful early epilepsy surgery. Epilepsia 51(7):1266–1276
44. Sadek A, Gray WP (2011) Chopping and changing: long-term results of epilepsy surgery. Lancet 378:1360–1362
45. Skirrow C et al (2011) Long-term intellectual outcome after temporal lobe surgery in childhood. Neurology 76(15):1330–1337
46. Spencer S, Huh L (2008) Outcomes of epilepsy surgery in adults and children. Lancet Neurol 7:525–537
47. Spencer SS et al (2002) Multiple subpial transection for intractable partial epilepsy: an international meta-analysis. Epilepsia 43(2):141–145
48. Thomas SG et al (2010) Cognitive changes following surgery in intractable hemispheric and sub-hemispheric pediatric epilepsy. Childs Nerv Syst 26:1067–1073
49. Weiner HL et al (2006) Epilepsy surgery in young children with tuberous sclerosis: results of a novel approach. Pediatrics 117(5):1494–1502
50. Wieser HG et al (2001) Proposal for a new classification of outcome with respect to epileptic seizures following epilepsy surgery. Epilepsia 42(2):282–286
51. Wyllie E et al (1988) Subdural electrodes in the evaluation for epilepsy surgery in children and adults. Neuropediatrics 19(2):80–86
52. Yoon HH et al (2003) Long-term seizure outcome in patients initially seizure-free after resective epilepsy surgery. Neurology 61(4):445–450

Magnetic Resonance Imaging in Epilepsy

Kader K. Oguz

Contents

Abstract With a major role in revealing epileptogenic lesions, magnetic resonance imaging (MRI) has also been very helpful in surgical planning and postoperative follow-up of drug-resistant focal epilepsies. In this article, in addition to discussing the most common epileptogenic lesions, advanced quantitative and functional MRI techniques in detecting abnormalities and revealing hemodynamic and microstructural changes are emphasized.

K.K. Oguz, M.D.
Faculty of Medicine, Hacettepe University,
06100, Sihhiye, Ankara, Turkey
e-mail: karlioguz@yahoo.com

N. Akalan, C. Di Rocco (eds.), *Pediatric Epilepsy Surgery*,
Advances and Technical Standards in Neurosurgery,
DOI 10.1007/978-3-7091-1360-8_3, © Springer-Verlag Wien 2012

Keywords Epilepsy • Magnetic Resonance Imaging • Functional • Diffusion Tensor Imaging • Seizure

Abbreviations

ASL	Arterial spin labeling
AVM	Arteriovenous malformation
BOLD	Blood oxygen level-dependent
CT	Computed tomography
DNET	Dysembryoplastic neuroepithelial tumor
DTI	Diffusion-tensor imaging
DWI	Diffusion-weighted imaging
ECS	Electrocortical stimulation
EEG	Electroencephalogram
FCD	Focal cortical dysplasia
FLAIR	Fluid-attenuated inversion recovery
fMRI	Functional magnetic resonance imaging
Gd	Gadolinium
GM	Gray matter
HS	Hippocampal sclerosis
IR	Inversion recovery
LGA	Low-grade astrocytoma
MCD	Malformation of cortical development
MPRAGE	Magnetization-prepared gradient-recalled echo
MRI	Magnetic resonance imaging
MRS	Magnetic resonance spectroscopy
MTC	Magnetization-transfer contrast
MTS	Mesial temporal sclerosis
PET	Fluorodeoxyglucose (FDG) positron emission tomography
PWI	Perfusion-weighted MR imaging
PXA	Pleomorphic xanthoastrocytoma
SE	Status epilepticus
SNR	Signal-to-noise ratio
SPECT	Single photon emission CT
SPGR	Spoiled gradient echo
SWI	Susceptibility-weighted imaging
TLE	Temporal lobe epilepsy
TSC	Tuberous sclerosis
VBM	Voxel-based morphometry
WM	White matter

Introduction

Among the modalities of neuroimaging, magnetic resonance imaging (MRI) has greatly impacted the management and outcome of patients with epilepsy. With a major role of revealing epileptogenic lesions, MRI has also been very helpful in the surgical planning and postoperative follow-up of drug-resistant focal epilepsies which constitute about 25 % of epilepsy cases. Although it is known that MRI in patients with idiopathic generalized epilepsy, benign rolandic epilepsy, and febrile seizures usually does not yield abnormalities but rather than ongoing epilepsy-related changes, the International League Against Epilepsy (ILAE) states that "Everybody with epilepsy should have, in the ideal situation, a high quality MRI!" Computed tomography (CT), once accepted as a first-line imaging modality, now is considered supplementary in the detection of calcification, as in cases of Sturge-Weber disease, tuberous sclerosis, or epileptogenic tumors.

Regardless of the underlying disease, patients in whom the lesions are visualized at preoperative MR imaging tend to have a better outcome after surgery for epilepsy than do patients without lesions [30, 45, 48].

In this article, in addition to discussing the most common lesions, advances in MRI and its potential in detecting abnormalities and revealing hemodynamic and microstuctural changes are emphasized.

Success of MRI in detecting abnormalities is determined by the scanner and applied techniques, the nature of the epileptogenic lesions, and the experience of the radiologist. One study found that the diagnostic yield of an MRI increases from 39 % with routine imaging interpreted by a general radiologist up to 90 % with an epilepsy-dedicated protocol interpreted by an experienced radiologist [68]. The radiologist should be experienced in epilepsy imaging and should assess the imaging with knowledge of the clinical semiology and electrophysiologic information (EEG).

Conventional MRI

An optimal MRI technique for detection of the epileptogenic lesion shows minor differences according to the patient's age. Due to maturing white matter, it can be more difficult to detect lesions and interpret them during first 24 months of life. While only T2-weighted (W) imaging should be replaced with that of minimum slice thickness without losing signal-to-noise ratio (SNR) in routine cranial MR imaging (which includes sagittal T1W and transverse and coronal T1W and T2W imaging in the author's institute) up to 8–10 months of age, addition of 3D T1 magnetization-prepared gradient-recalled echo (MPRAGE) or spoiled gradient echo (SPGR) with a 1–1.5 mm slice thickness is necessary from 8–10 to 24–30 months. These sequences provide a good gray-white matter contrast at this stage of myelination. Afterward, epilepsy-dedicated MRI protocol does not differ from that of adults: Adult protocol differs from pediatric cases older than 24–30 months in that it should include coronal high-resolution T2W and inversion recovery (IR) slices with a 2–3-mm thickness oriented perpendicular to the hippocampi, especially in cases of temporal lobe epilepsy (TLE) [3]. In patients with a history or suspicion of trauma or a vascular lesion, a more definitive diagnosis can be achieved by adding T2* gradient echo or susceptibility-weighted imaging (SWI) to the protocol, depending on the facility [55].

Gadolinium (Gd)-based contrast materials should be considered when the radiologist or technician comes across a tumor or tumor-like lesion to get a more specific differential diagnosis or to plan the surgery. Additionally, intravenous contrast materials can be used in dynamic-enhanced susceptibility-weighted perfusion imaging to supplement other techniques such as evaluation of peri-ictal hemodynamic changes or determination of the extent of the pial angiomas in Sturge-Weber syndrome [49, 56].

Neuroimaging of Common Epileptogenic Substrates

Although epileptogenic substrates are practically the same in children and adults, their proportion changes, i.e., malformation of cortical development and developmental tumors are more common in children and young adults while hippocampal sclerosis is more common in adults [17] .

Epilepsy-Associated Tumors

Epilepsy-associated tumors are slow-growing, well-defined, non-necrotic lesions that develop from the cortex and do have a common association with malformation of cortical development. Clinical presentation in seizures and complete surgical removal of these lesions result in successful seizure control [50].

Images of these tumors have common features: a cortical well-defined lesion, no accompanying edema or necrosis, and a scalloped/remodeled adjacent bone due to the tumor's long-term presence. Most critical radiological points of evaluation include its location, detection of associated focal cortical dysplasia (FCD), presence of calcification and cyst, and enhancement. Once an epilepsy-associated tumor is detected, one should also search for hippocampal sclerosis because it is common in double pathologies in epilepsy patients [18, 19].

Gangliogliomas and Gangliocytomas

Gangliomas are more frequent (approximately ten times) and bigger in macroscopic size in children than in adults [11, 60]. The usual location is the temporal lobe with a

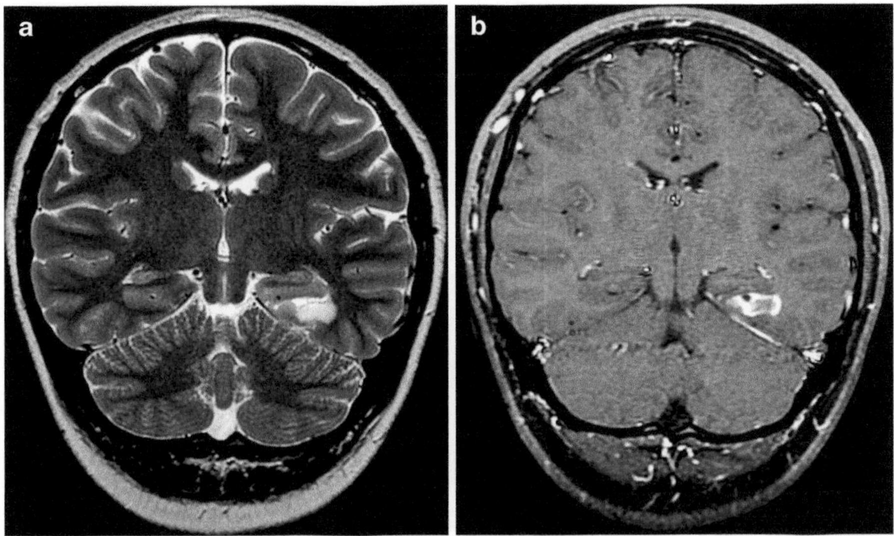

Fig. 1 Ganglioglioma in the left temporal lobe. Bright cortical lesion on T2W imaging (**a**) shows enhancement on postcontrast T1W imaging (**b**)

mild predilection for the mesial surface. Together with low-grade astrocytomas, they are the most common tumors in temporal lobectomy specimens [7]. Because they can present as a cyst, a solid mass, or a mixture of both, their density on CT varies, with about 30–50 % calcification. Usually they are hypointense, sometimes having an internal mild hyperintensity on T1-W series of MRI and hyperintensity on T2-W imaging unless they have a concretion, which gives a dark appearance. Approximately half of them enhance either in a nodular, solid, or peripheral pattern [46] (Fig. 1a, b).

Different from gangliogliomas, which consist of neuronal and glial cells, gangliocytomas histologically consist of only neurons and are rarely seen. These lesions usually have solid and cystic components and show enhancement on post-Gd T1-W series.

Dysembryoplastic Neuroepithelial Tumors (DNET)

These are wedge-shaped tumors with a temporal and frontal lobe predominance and frequently coexist with FCDs DNET are commonly missed or invisible on MRI. They are characterized by a "tail" toward the ventricles, "bubbly" appearance due to a well-marginated multilobulated configuration, and very high T2 and low T1 signal intensities [16, 31] (Fig. 2a, b). Fluid-attenuated inversion-recovery (FLAIR) sequence gives invaluable information about their differential diagnosis from other cortical tumors. First, DNETs are proven to be "pseudocystic" because they have a high signal on FLAIR, which shows their solid nature, in contrast to their "cystic" signals on T1- and T2-W imaging. Second, a thin peripheral bright rim on FLAIR imaging has been reported to be pathognomonic of DNETs [59]. Although a classic DNET does not enhance, a faint, punctate, or rim enhancement can be seen in some

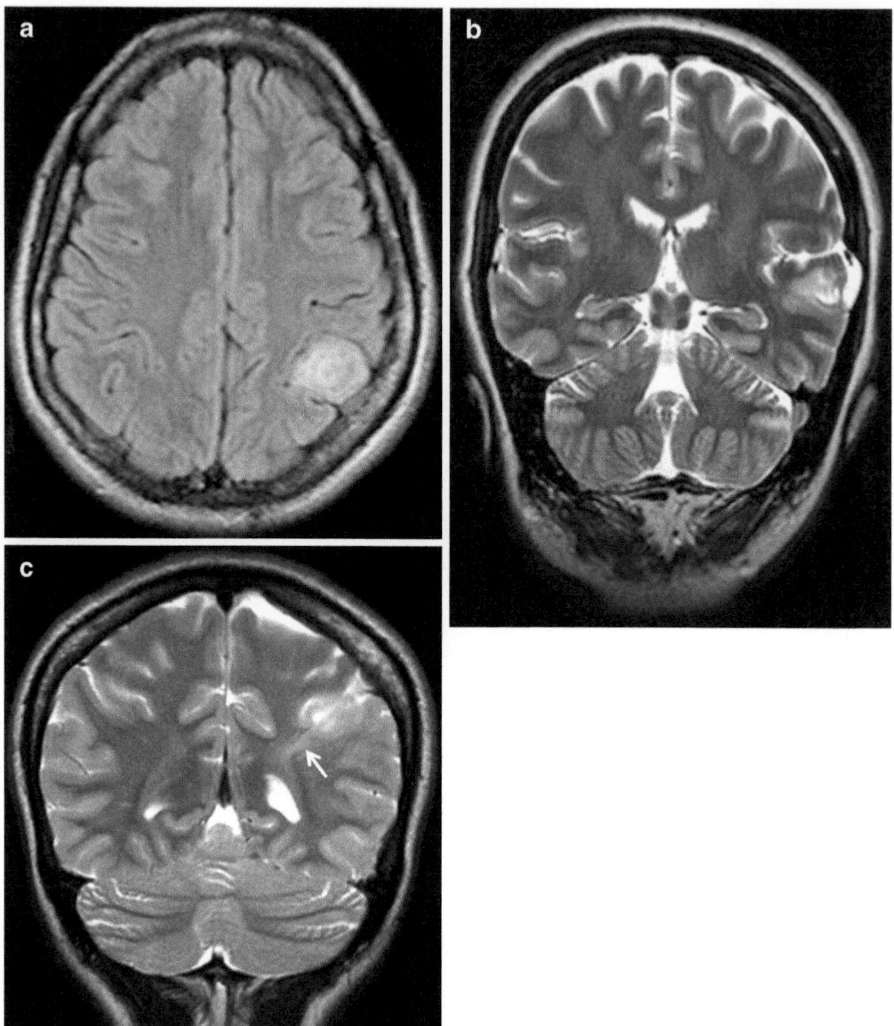

Fig. 2 (**a**) A DNET in the left parietal lobe appears as a hyperintense, rounded, well-defined cortical mass without peripheral edema on an axial FLAIR image. (**b**) Another DNET is seen in the left temporal lobe on a coronal T2W image. Note the prominent hyperintensity and remodeled thin adjacent bone as a result of the tumor's longstanding presence. (**c**) A tail toward the ventricle (*arrow*) can be seen

cases. A tail extending to the ventricles can also be observed in cortical tubers and FCD with balloon cells (Fig. 2c). DNETs usually remain stable in size; however, seizures may continue despite multiple antiepileptic drug regimens. An MRI for unsuccessful seizure control following surgery should be performed, with the protocol dedicated to epilepsy (as described in the previous section). The radiologist

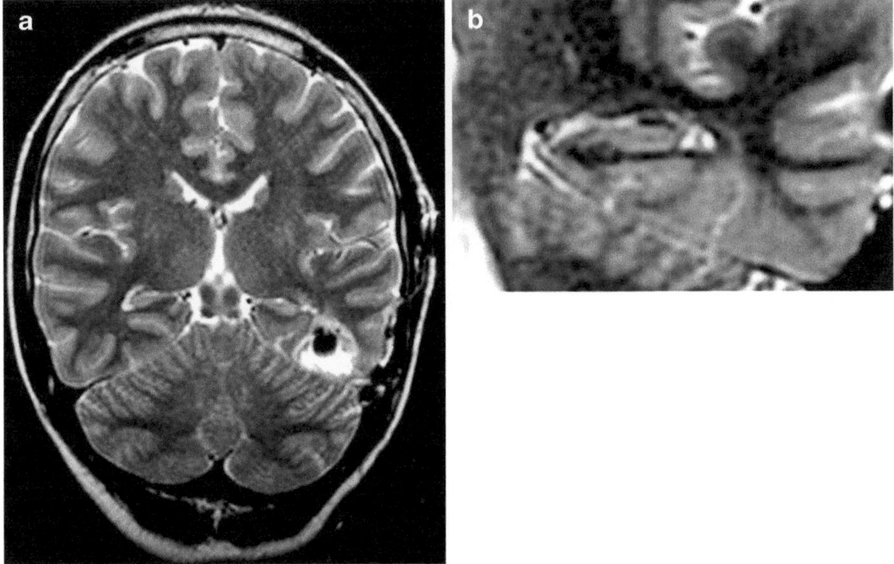

Fig. 3 (**a**) Coronal T2W image obtained immediately after resection of a DNET (not shown, scanned in another institution) from the left temporal lobe in a 12-year-old boy shows acute hemorrhage in the operation bed as profound hypointensity. As a result of uncontrolled seizures following surgery, another MRI was obtained 2 years later. (**b**) High-resolution T2-W TSE coronal image shows increased cortical thickness and blurred white-gray-matter junction suggestive of cortical dysplasia

should look for an incomplete resection of the tumor and/or a previously missed associated cortical dysplasia [61] (Fig. 3a, b). The latter is more common when preoperative MRI is performed routinely or with imaging sequences having poorer resolution.

Pleomorphic Xanthoastrocytomas

As common features with other epilepsy-associated tumors, pleomorphic xanthoastrocytomas (PXAs) affect predominantly the supratentorial compartment, and most commonly the temporal lobe followed by the frontal lobe cortex. These tumors also show solid and deeper cystic portions and, thus, solid and deeper signal intensities on MRI. Peripheral cortical location, solid enhancing nodule, and continuity with enhancing dura (tail) are well known features of PXAs. Usually no calcification is seen on CT and no perilesional edema is observed [32, 41]. They share common radiologic features with desmoplastic infantile ganglioglioma; however, PXAs usually present in the second decade or around late childhood. A close association with FCD in adjacent cortex should be considered during evaluation [47].

Low-Grade Astrocytomas

MRI is more successful in detecting these cortical, infiltrative, ill-defined masses. Low-grade astrocytomas (LGAs) do not enhance. When present, a more aggressive/anaplastic form should be suspected. Expansion of the cortex, which is commonly the frontal and temporal lobes, is usual but not the rule. Thus, sometimes it is necessary to perform a follow-up MRI or add diffusion-weighted imaging (DWI) or magnetic resonance spectroscopy (MRS) to differentiate these lesions from FCDs, infarcts, and encephalitis radiologically. Valuable information comes from the history and clinical findings of the patient and usually solves the problem.

Rarer epilepsy-associated tumors will not be mentioned here because of their nonspecific radiological findings.

Hippocampal Sclerosis

Mesial temporal sclerosis (MTS) or hippocampal sclerosis (HS) occurs from pyramidal and neuronal cell loss in the cornu ammonis and dentate of the hippocampus. It is not only the most frequent epilepsy substrate in patients undergoing surgery for epilepsy, but also the most frequent cause of complex partial seizures in adults [52]. Patients often have a history of complicated febrile seizures during childhood [26, 67]. A familial tendency of mesial temporal lobe epilepsy has been reported [25, 36]. Currently, the most preferred surgical procedure for treatment is the anterior temporal lobectomy [17, 35].

Three major findings that should suggest HS can easily be evaluated on coronal thin section (2–3 mm) T2W imaging acquired perpendicular to the hippocampi. These are atrophy, T2 signal increase, and loss of internal structure of the hippocampus (Fig. 4). Inversion recovery sequences help determine internal structure of a hippocampus [13, 14]. Supplementary MRI findings, such as loss of ipsilateral pes hippocampus digitations, decreased thickness of the collateral white matter, and dilatation of the ipsilateral temporal horn of the lateral ventricle, usually occur secondary to hippocampal involvement. Other MRI abnormalities result from degeneration through the components of the Papez circuit and include atrophy of the ipsilateral fornix and mammillary body (Fig. 4) [20]. Increased signal intensity of the ipsilateral anterior temporal lobe white matter and loss of the gray-white-matter boundary are often seen and can be due to degeneration and myelin loss or associated malformation of cortical development [54]. Involvement of the amygdala, which is usually indicated by a subtle increase in the T2 signal and a volume change, should be reported for prognostic importance because isolated HS has a better outcome after surgery [15].

An experienced radiologist can recognize HS with a sensitivity of 80–90 %. However, in bilateral cases (10–20 %) [38] or in cases without a visible radiologic abnormality, quantitative assessment such as MR volumetry and T2 relaxation measurements or use of more advanced techniques such as magnetization-transfer contrast (MTC), MRS, and diffusion-tensor imaging (DTI) may be necessary. A quantitative approach, however, requires extra energy, trained personnel, software, and time, all of

Fig. 4 Coronal T2W TSE image shows atrophy and hyperintensity of the left hippocampus, suggestive of hippocampal sclerosis (*white arrow*). Note the dilated ipsilateral temporal horn, decreased thickness of the collateral white matter, and atrophy of the ipsilateral mammillary body (*black arrow*)

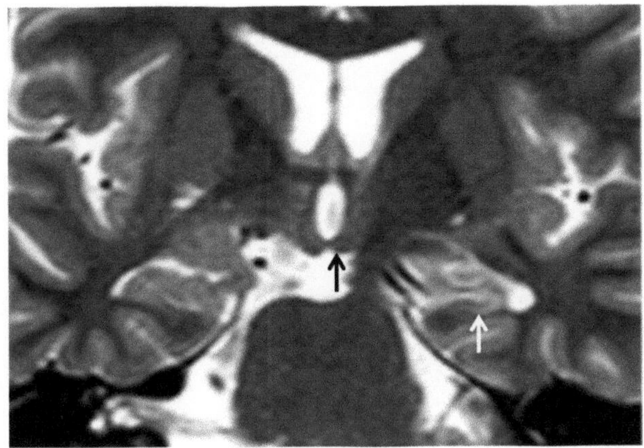

which are especially precious to busy radiology departments. Volume loss has been found to correlate with the duration of epileptic disorder, frequency of childhood febrile seizures, memory function, and cell loss on pathological examinations [21, 24]. A literature review by Keller and Roberts [44] summarized brain changes that occur in temporal lobe epilepsy (TLE) patients revealed by a total of 18 voxel-based morphometry (VBM) studies. In this fully automated quantitative technique, gray matter concentration and volume are measured via voxel-wise statistical analyses. Following a series of preprocessing steps, i.e., spatial normalization, tissue segmentation, and spatial smoothing in standard fashion, morphologic differences are detected in two groups of people [2]. Bilateral asymmetric widespread abnormalities occur preferentially ipsilateral to the side of seizure focus. These structures include hippocampus, amygdala, parahippocampal gyrus, entorhinal and perirhinal cortexes, fusiform gyrus, temporal pole, superior, middle, and inferior temporal gyri, fornix, orbital frontal lobe, frontal pole, insula, parietal lobe, and cingulated gyrus. White matter (WM) reductions also occur in predominantly ipsilateral temporal and extratemporal lobes, although VBM is not the technique of choice for evaluating WM due to insufficient WM tracts for effective spatial normalization. Additionally, some studies found an increase in gray matter (GM) concentration mostly in the temporal lobe. However, a parallel increase in volume of GM was not observed. Although this remains speculative, the frequent coexistence of malformation of cortical development (MCD), observed as blurred gray-to-white-matter [53] transition on MRI, can manifest as increased GM concentration or displacement of the parahippocampal gyrus due to severe atrophy [43].

Malformation of Cortical Development

Malformation of cortical development lesions and their imaging should be discussed in a separate article on migration disorders. However, two lesions that undergo surgical resection or other types of surgical procedures are discussed here: FCDs and tuberous sclerosis.

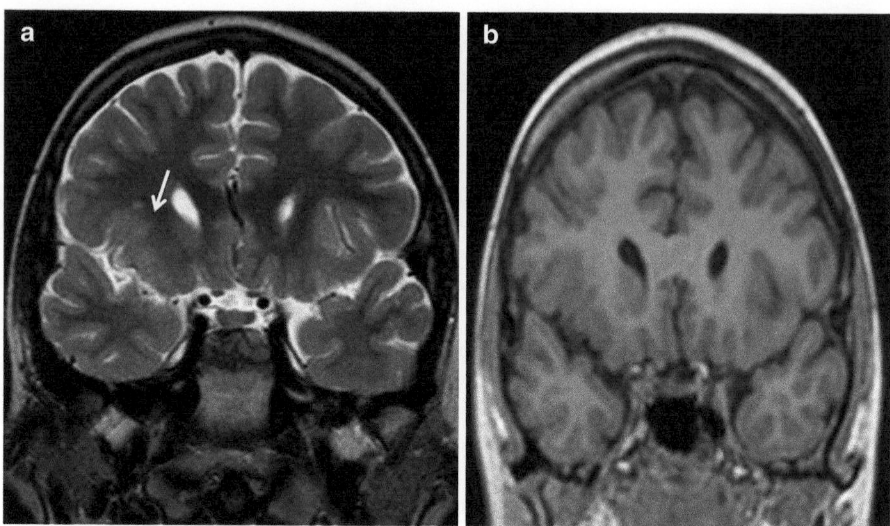

Fig. 5 A frontal cortical dysplasia is apparent sometimes only on the thin-slice coronal images. This is such an example. Coronal T2W TSE (*arrow*, **a**) and coronal T1W 3D SPGR (**b**) images show thick cortex and blurring at the gray-to-white-matter transition with a small subcortical heterotopias beneath

Focal Cortical Dysplasia

Since its initial description by Taylor et al. [65], FCDs have been extensively studied and classified and refer to a wide range of cortical formation abnormalities. Classification of FCDs based on the neuropathological findings by Palmini et al. in 2004 has been widely accepted and used [58]. However, in 2011, the ILAE task force developed a new classification system to distinguish isolated forms (FCD types I and II) from those associated with another principal lesion (FCD type III) [12]. While mild FCD usually shows no visible radiologic abnormality, as suggested by Palmini et al., a subtle increase in the T2 signal and hypoplasia of mostly the temporal lobe with type 1A and 1B can be seen. The usual findings of a FCD include thick cortex, blurring of the gray-to-white-matter transition, abnormally increased signal in the subjacent white matter, and deep and asymmetric abnormal sulci (Fig. 5a, b) [51]. Broadening of the gyri with increased T2 signal and accompanying "tail" tapering toward the ventricle [23, 66] have been accepted characteristics of type 2B (FCD with balloon cells) (Fig. 6). Keeping mild FCD types 1 and 2 suggested by Palmini et al., this new classification by the ILAE task force took those FCDs plus adjacent HS (a), glial/glioneural tumor (b), vascular malformation (c), or lesions acquired early in life such as trauma, ischemic sequela, encephalitis (d) into consideration (Fig. 7) [12]. However, a rare association between FCD type 2 and these entities within different locations of the brain parenchyma is not considered FCD type 3. FCD type 3a, which indicates FCD in an adjacent parenchyma and HS, should be

Fig. 6 A right frontal cortical dysplasia of type 2B (with balloon cells) with expansion of the gyri and a faint tail toward the lateral ventricle is seen on the coronal T2W TSE image

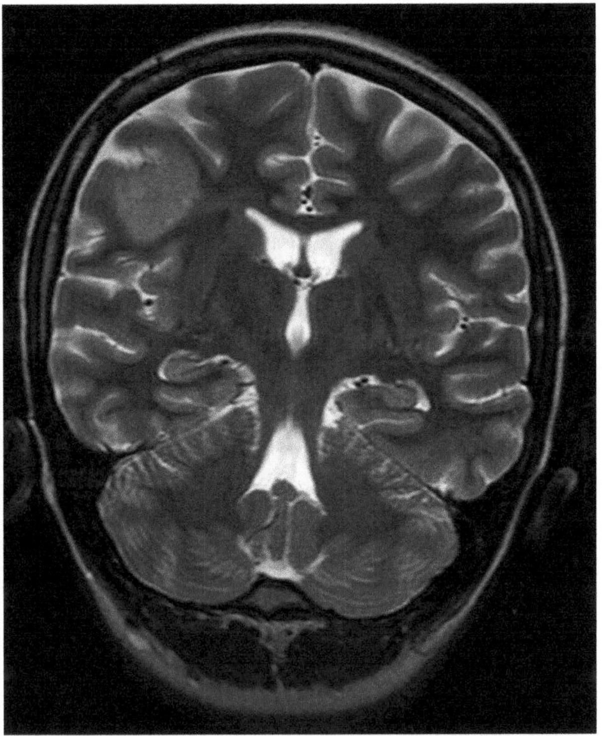

differentiated from "double" and "dual pathology" terms. In cases without HS, the presence of two epileptogenic lesions is defined as "double pathology," while HS plus an extratemporal lesion is defined as "dual pathology" (Fig. 8a, b). Since dual pathology is observed in approximately 15 % of the patients with HS, one should always search for abnormalities in addition to HS [18].

Tuberous Sclerosis

Multiple cortical and subcortical tubers and subependymal nodules along the lateral ventricles are characteristic features of tuberous sclerosis (TSC). Tubers expand the gyri they originate and cause an increased T2 signal in the cortex and subjacent white matter. When there is calcification, the signal can differ, i.e., a lower T2 signal and a higher T1 signal. Subependymal nodules usually are calcified and seen as T1 hyper- and T2 hypointense nodules (Fig. 9a). They can be observed along the ventricles on 3D MPRAGE/SPGR images, even when they are in the submillimeter size range. The similar radiologic appearance of a cortical tuber and that of a FCD with balloon cells or a DNET leads one to consider TSC as a "syndromic variant" of FCD or that they all have a common precursor cell (Fig. 9b) [37]. From a radiologic point of view, multiplicity of the tubers and the presence of subependymal nodules

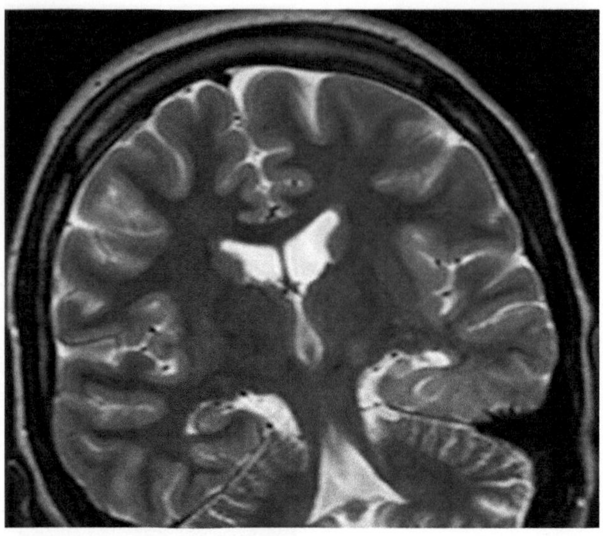

Fig. 7 Left hippocampal sclerosis associated with adjacent temporal cortical dysplasia can be classified as type III A

help in the diagnosis of TSC. Early in life, due to the lack of myelin, recognition of a tuber may be difficult. Thus, T1W imaging is a most valuable sequence with hyperintensity of these lesions (Fig. 10a, b) [4].

Patients with TSC frequently are not candidates for epilepsy surgery because of multiplicity of the lesions and types of seizures. However, when electrophysiology and imaging with single photon emission computed tomography (SPECT), along with the seizures that the patient experiences, indicate a specific focus, then surgery is considered.

Other

Cavernomas are best depicted on T2*GRE, SWI, but their internal structure, with its multiple phases of blood products and dark hemosiderin periphery, is usually seen on T1- and T2W series (Fig. 11a, b). These cortical and juxtacortical lesions are highly epileptogenic and are not difficult to diagnose radiologically unless they are huge and complicated with recent hemorrhage.

Arteriovenous malformations (AVMs) with their tangle of vessels, large feeding and draining vasculature, and accompanying aneurysm usually pose no diagnostic challenge.

'Similarly, with characteristic CT and MRI findings of Sturge-Weber Syndrome such as calcification of subcortical parenchyma which are affected by overlying pial angiomas, asymmetric atrophy of the parenchyma most frequently parietal and occipital lobes, enlarged ipsilateral choroid plexus and linear superficial enhancement with Gd, diagnosis of this syndrome is straight forward (Fig. 12a, b).

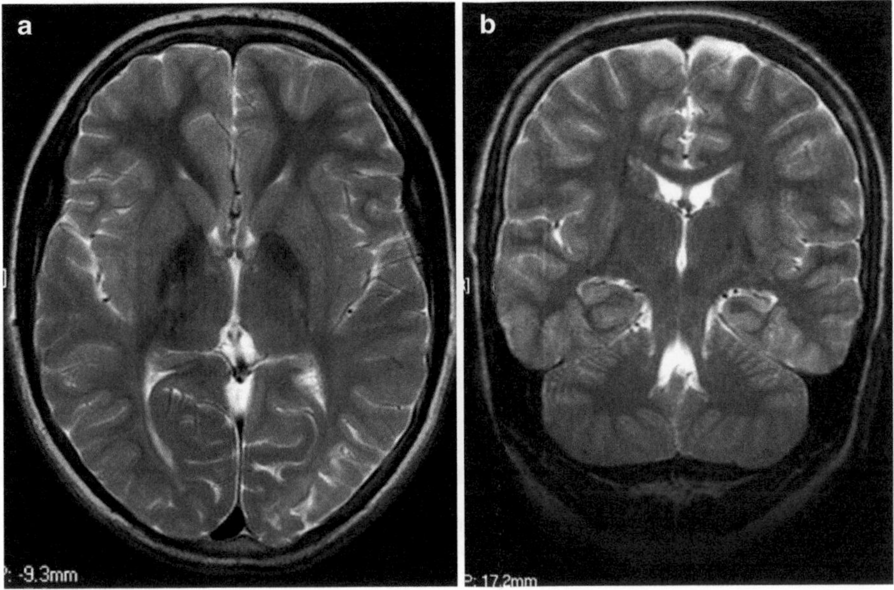

Fig. 8 (**a**) Axial T2W image of left occipital sequela seen as parenchymal loss in a 7-year-old girl. (**b**) Coronal T2W image shows left hippocampal sclerosis with atrophy and increased signal. A dual pathology is found in about 15 % of HS patients

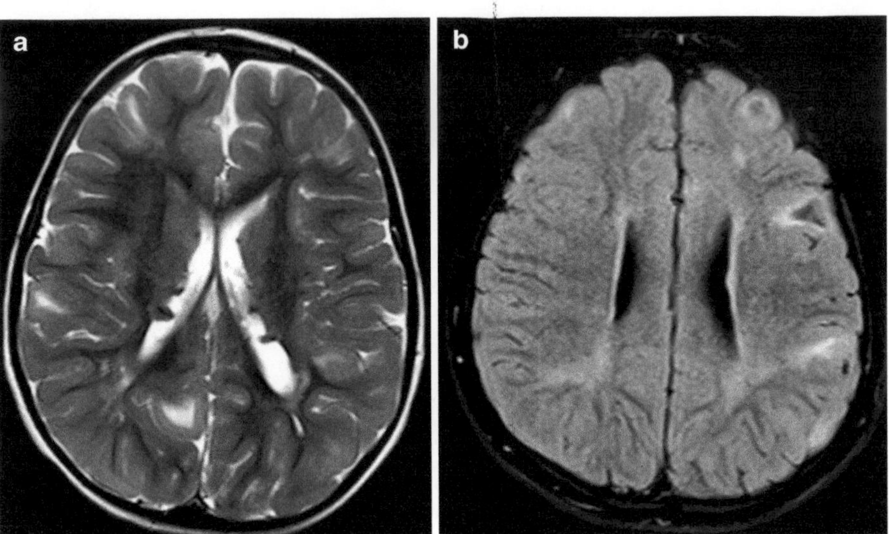

Fig. 9 MR imaging of two patients with tuberous sclerosis. (**a**) T2-hypointense subependymal nodules and T2-hyperintense cortical tubers. (**b**) FLAIR image shows tails of the tubers extending to the ventricles

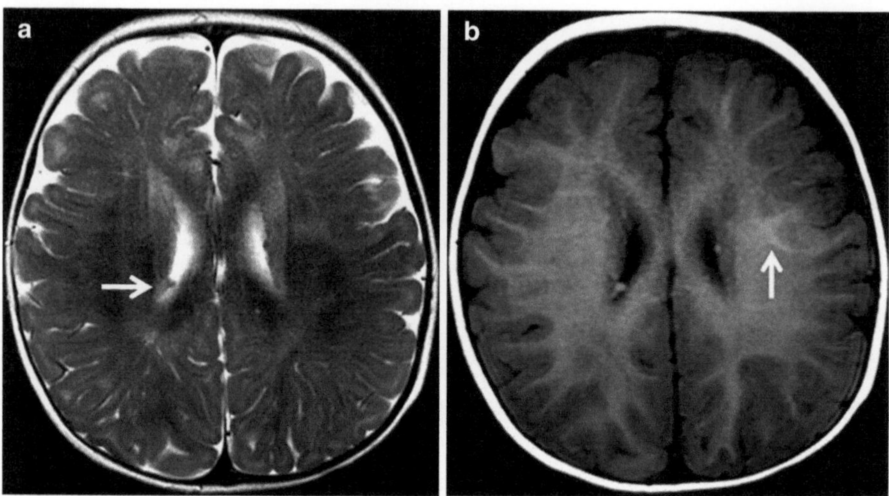

Fig. 10 (**a**) T2W image of a 7 month-old infant with seizures; faint cortical tubers are hardly seen with well-described subependymal nodules (*arrow*). (**b**) T1W image in which the "tails" of the tubers can be recognized by their hyperintensity (*arrow*)

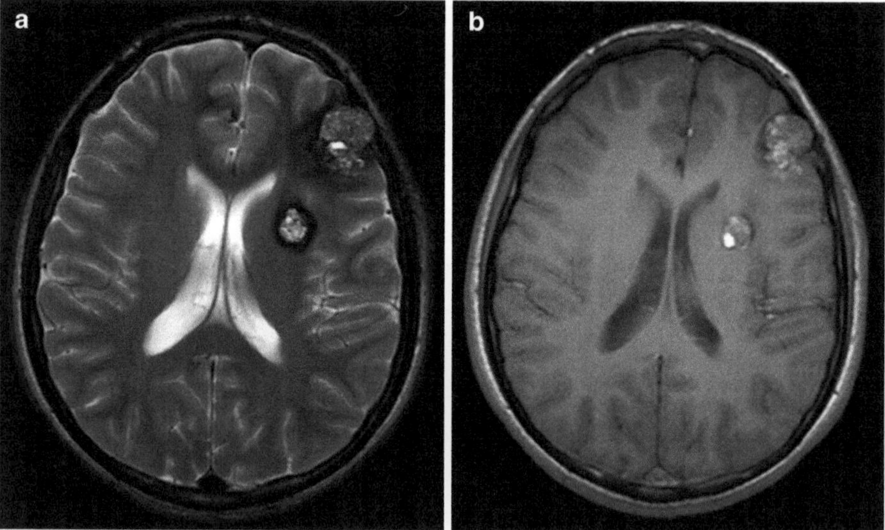

Fig. 11 Multiple cavernomas with peripheral complete hemosiderin dark rim and bright internal core are seen on axial T2W (**a**) and T1W (**b**) views of a 14-year-old boy

Determining the regions of the affected brain may be more challenging than diagnosis. SPECT, PET, and perfusion-weighted MR imaging can delineate hemodynamically and metabolically abnormal areas in candidates for surgery, especially because involvement of other hemisphere becomes important.

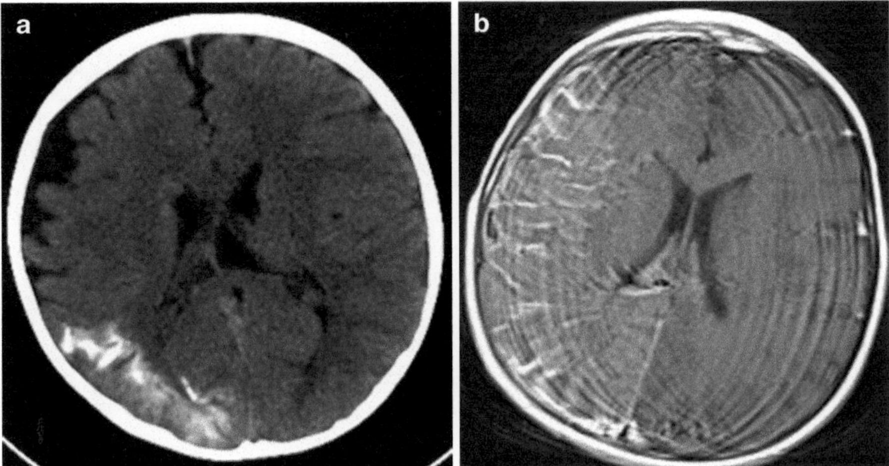

Fig. 12 CT (**a**) and MR imaging (**b**) of a patient with Sturge-Weber syndrome show profound subcortical calcification and linear enhancement of widespread pial angiomas on postcontrast T1W imaging

Status Epilepticus

During the peri-ictal phase of status epilepticus (SE), regional cortical changes and remote lesions, including cerebellar diaschisis, ipsilateral thalamic lesions, and basal ganglia lesions, have been reported. These lesions are observed as tissue swelling, hyperintensity most prominent on FLAIR imaging, and restricted diffusion (Fig. 13a, b) [39]. Peri-ictal radiologic findings are usually reversible, and these abnormalities may reflect the real extent of epileptogenic activity. Later sequelae, including focal brain atrophy, cortical laminar necrosis, and mesial temporal sclerosis, can occur. Thalamic DWI hyperintense lesions, occurring after prolonged partial SE, have received attention recently and probably represent participation of the thalamus in the propagation of partial seizures in SE because of reciprocal connections with the involved cortex (Fig. 13b) [39, 42]. Gd enhancement may occur in the hippocampi, which may be followed by sclerosis (Fig.14a, b). Diffusion restriction as shown by reduced ADC in the hippocampi, the pulvinar region of the thalamus, and cortical regions may give correlates of hyperperfusion assessed by SPECT or perfusion-weighted MR imaging (PWI) [63].

Cryptogenic Epilepsy

Although prolonged EEG recordings with intracranial electrodes have increased the success in resecting the epileptogenic cortex, because of complications of this procedure and the possibility of removing the electrodes without identifying the seizure focus,

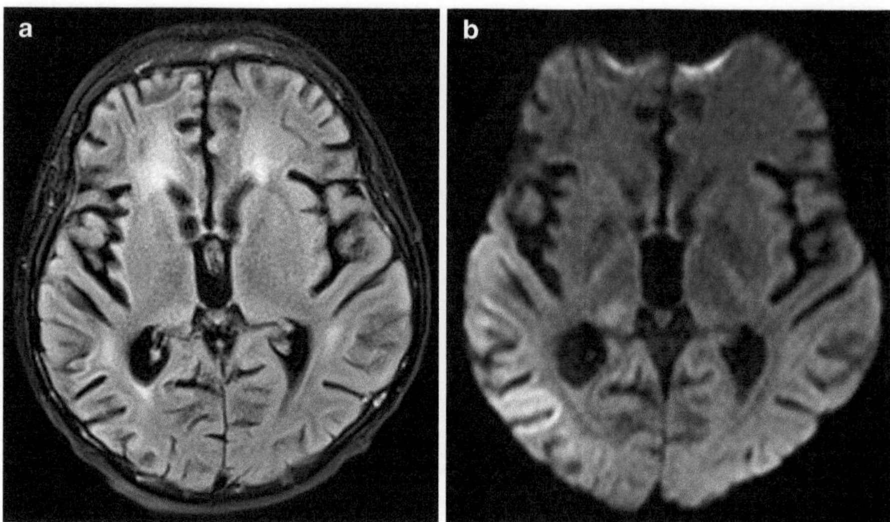

Fig. 13 Peri-ictal FLAIR (**a**) and DWI (**b**) images show increased signals suggestive of cytotoxic edema assessed by DWI in temporo-occipital cortices as well as the ipsilateral pulvinar of the thalamus

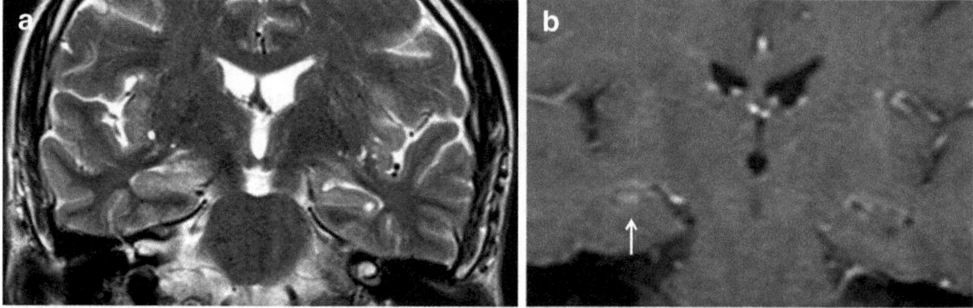

Fig. 14 Peri-ictal changes in the right hippocampus: swelling and T2 hyperintensity on the T2W image (**a**) and contrast enhancement on the postcontrast T1W image (*arrow*, **b**)

surgery in the absence of a visible MR lesion continues to be a challenge. As imaging techniques and their diagnostic yield improve, previously accepted "cryptogenic" epilepsies may turn out to be "lesional" [9]. The most common histopathological finding in cryptogenic epilepsy is focal cortical dysplasia. High magnetic field systems and phase-array coils will enable detection and delineation of malformed areas and, in turn, increase the number of patients who will benefit from surgery. T1W volumetric acquisition with isotropic 1-mm^3 voxels not only increases the visibility of the lesions, it also provides multiplanar reformats. Curvilinear reformatting in particular decreases artifactual cortical thickening and increases the detection of these abnormalities [6, 40].

Voxel-based morphometry (VBM) is a technique that enables identification of regional differences in the whole brain through a multiple-step process. However, it is time consuming to perform, and subtle increased cortical thickness due to cortical reorganization from personal abilities and specifications and prominent signal changes of the lesions may lead to confusion and reduced sensitivity [22]. Histopathological correlation of findings obtained from VBM is needed. Besides VBM and T2-relaxivity measurements, DTI, by quantifying diffusivity of water, adds information about the microstructure of brain tissue [33, 51]. DTI revealed abnormalities in white matter adjacent to and often beyond the cortical dysplasia [28, 69]. TLE patients, as discussed in the relevant section of this chapter, show widespread diffusion abnormality in white matter [33].

Since blood oxygen level-dependent (BOLD) imaging can detect local changes in oxy- and deoxyhemoglobin concentrations due to neuronal activity related to epileptic discharge, combined EEG and fMRI studies, coregistered with anatomical data, can reveal an epileptic zone [34].

In addition to dynamic susceptibility-weighted perfusion imaging, another technique recently available in the market, "Arterial Spin Labeling" (ASL), gives information comparable to that of single photon emission computed tomography (SPECT). An advantage of ASL is that it quantifies cerebral blood flow. If by chance the patient is not having a seizure during the MR examination, ASL will disclose interictal abnormalities. Adding ASL may provide additional information about the lateralization of the focus [51, 71]. 18-Fluorodeoxyglucose (FDG) positron emission tomography (PET) is especially helpful in lateralization of the focus by showing interictal hypometabolism. The focus may actually be at the site of margin [51]. Coregistration of PET data with volumetric T1W imaging overcomes the poor resolution of this technique.

Although these advanced imaging techniques can provide valuable information about the epileptogenic zone, currently no single technique is capable of delineating the exact extent of cortical lesions. Further studies with correlation between disciplines, including histopathology and immunohistochemistry, are necessary to determine the clinical significance of these imaging findings.

Functional MR (fMR) Imaging

Among advanced MR imaging modalities, fMR imaging merits special attention. This technique relies on a signal that arises from the oxygenation status of hemoglobin, the so-called BOLD signal. Close correlation of neural activity and changes in tissue oxygen level enable visualization of the BOLD signal. A block (alternating active and baseline cycles) or event-related (discrete unequal events) paradigm is present; however, under clinical circumstances a block-design paradigm provides a higher signal-to-noise ratio and decreases the scan time necessary for robust fMR imaging activation. fMR studies are performed in epilepsy patients for two reasons: to evaluate the relationship of a lesion with eloquent cortex and to assess hemispheric dominance (Fig. 15). A variety of tasks may be used; however, this poses a problem in standardization of the technique and the results obtained from studies. For expressive language, frequently silent word generation from letters or words is used.

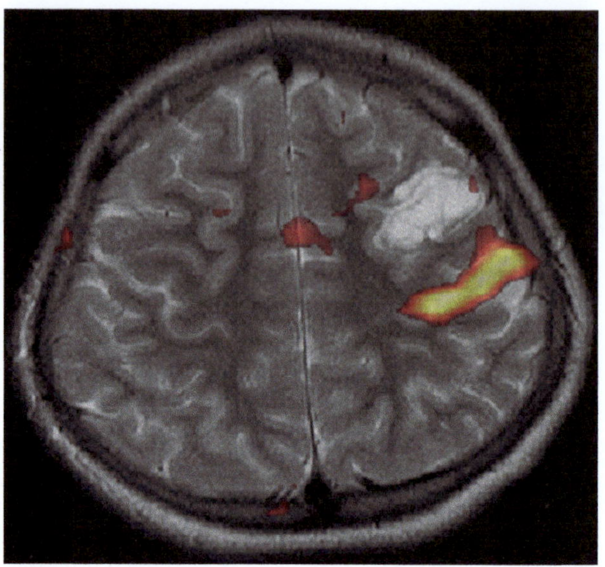

Fig. 15 fMRI study of a right-hand motor task shows BOLD activation at one gyrus beyond the right frontal DNET

Because of the increased frequency of right-sided or bilateral language, lateralization or intrahemispheric reorganization can occur in patients with left hemisphere lesions [1, 17, 27], and an intracarotid amobarbital test (Wada test) or, increasingly, fMRI is performed to assess the language/speech deficit risks of the surgery [5, 64]. Up to 90 % of cases studied found agreement between these techniques [8, 29, 70] and even found fMR imaging to be a better predictor of postoperative cognitive outcome [10, 62]. It has been emphasized that at least three different language tasks of sufficient length and the combination of electrocortical stimulation (ECS) and fMR imaging should be obtained. fMR imaging should be performed by a technician/radiologist with expertise and be interpreted with special attention paid to the individual's task performance and the extent of cluster size of the BOLD signal on postprocessing . fMR imaging has advantages over ECS: atypical locations of eloquent cortex can be detected by imaging. Although fMR imaging cannot replace ECS or WADA completely, it decreases the need for these invasive tests and helps in planning surgical strategy and the targeting of sites for ECS.

Fiber tractography showing 3D orientation of white matter tracts in combination with fMR imaging enables the surgeon to assess the relationship between the lesion and the WM bundle and eloquent cortex simultaneously (Fig. 16a–c).

Postoperative Imaging

Evaluation of a postoperative MR study necessitates knowledge of the surgery performed, its potential complications, and previous epileptogenic lesion characteristics if

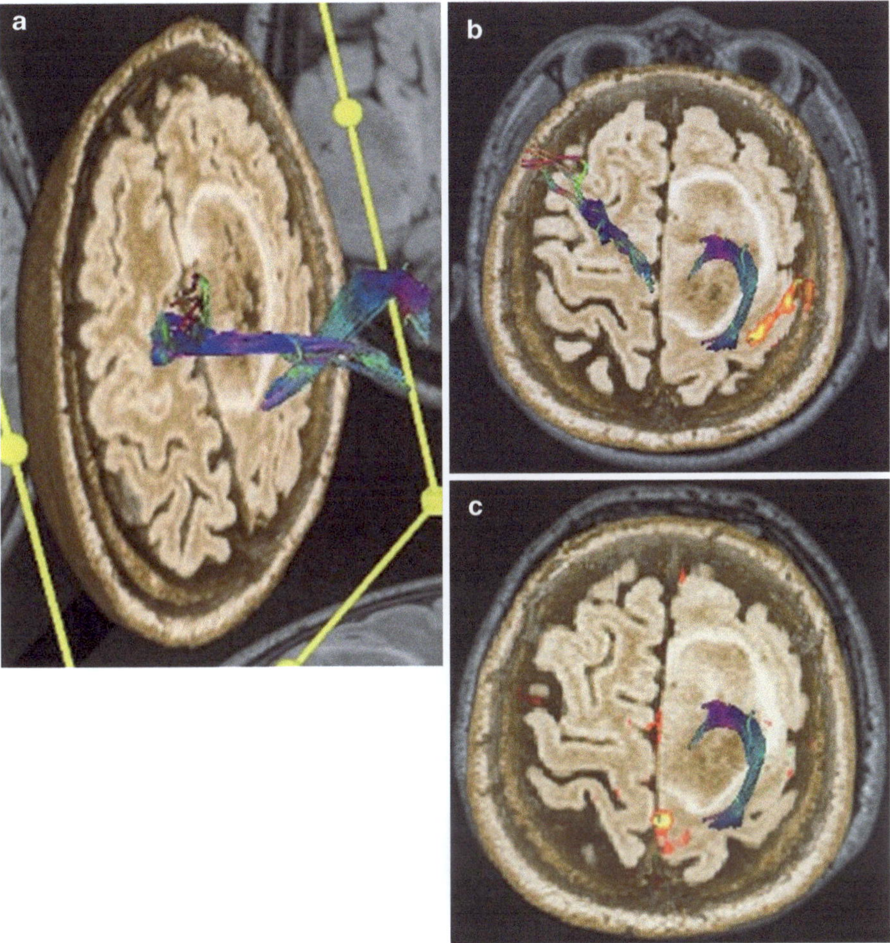

Fig. 16 Fiber tractography of the corticospinal tractus (*CST*) coregistered with FLAIR imaging (**a**) shows posterior displacement of the left CST by the tumor. BOLD activation from right-hand (**b**) and right-foot (**c**) motor tasks shows posterolateral (**b**) and posteromedial (**c**) deviation of the activation by the mass

visible on MR imaging. Local postsurgical changes include hemorrhage and cytotoxic tissue edema displayed b`y DWI, and sometimes infarcts in arterial territory similar to those in other cranial operations [57]. MR imaging protocol should be planned with knowledge of the preoperative imaging findings, i.e., epilepsy protocol in FCD, contrast-enhanced routine imaging in neoplastic lesions, and contrast-enhanced imaging, including thin-section T2W imaging perpendicular to the temporal lobe developmental tumors.

In patients who were operated on but not seizure-free, a repeat MR imaging procedure should be performed if a higher magnetic field system and newer imaging modalities with higher resolution become available.

Conclusion

Patients with drug-resistant epilepsy benefit from advances in imaging for the localization and lateralization of epileptogenic substrate and the planning of surgery in cryptogenic and lesional epilepsy. MR imaging provides information about hemodynamic and microstructural tissue properties as well. Once overlooked subtle cortical dysplasias will probably be captured via developing quantitative and functional imaging techniques in the near future.

References

1. Anderson DP, Harvey AS, Saling MM, Anderson V, Kean M, Abbott DF, Wellard RM, Jackson GD (2006) FMRI lateralization of expressive language in children with cerebral lesions. Epilepsia 47(6):998–1008
2. Ashburner J, Friston KJ (2000) Voxel-based morphometry – the methods. Neuroimage 11 (6 Pt 1):805–821
3. Atlas SW (2009) Magnetic resonance imaging of the brain and spine, 4th edn. Lippincott Williams & Wilkins, Philadelphia, pp 312–313
4. Baron Y, Barkovich AJ (1999) MR imaging of tuberous sclerosis in neonates and young infants. AJNR Am J Neuroradiol 20(5):907–916
5. Bargalló N (2008) Functional magnetic resonance: new applications in epilepsy. Eur J Radiol 67(3):401–408
6. Bastos AC, Comeau RM, Andermann F, Melanson D, Cendes F, Dubeau F, Fontaine S, Tampieri D, Olivier A (1999) Diagnosis of subtle focal dysplastic lesions: curvilinear reformatting from three-dimensional magnetic resonance imaging. Ann Neurol 46(1):88–94
7. Benifla M, Otsubo H, Ochi A, Weiss SK, Donner EJ, Shroff M, Chuang S, Hawkins C, Drake JM, Elliott I, Smith ML, Snead OC 3rd, Rutka JT (2006) Temporal lobe surgery for intractable epilepsy in children: an analysis of outcomes in 126 children. Neurosurgery 59(6): 1203–1213
8. Benke T, Köylü B, Visani P, Karner E, Brenneis C, Bartha L, Trinka E, Trieb T, Felber S, Bauer G, Chemelli A, Willmes K (2006) Language lateralization in temporal lobe epilepsy: a comparison between fMRI and the Wada Test. Epilepsia 47(8):1308–1319
9. Bernasconi A, Bernasconi N, Bernhardt BC, Schrader D (2011) Advances in MRI for 'cryptogenic' epilepsies. Nat Rev Neurol 7(2):99–108
10. Binder JR, Sabsevitz DS, Swanson SJ, Hammeke TA, Raghavan M, Mueller WM (2008) Use of preoperative functional MRI to predict verbal memory decline after temporal lobe epilepsy surgery. Epilepsia 49(8):1377–1394
11. Blümcke I, Löbach M, Wolf HK, Wiestler OD (1999) Evidence for developmental precursor lesions in epilepsy-associated glioneuronal tumors. Microsc Res Tech 46(1):53–58
12. Blümcke I, Thom M, Aronica E, Armstrong DD, Vinters HV, Palmini A, Jacques TS, Avanzini G, Barkovich AJ, Battaglia G, Becker A, Cepeda C, Cendes F, Colombo N, Crino P, Cross JH, Delalande O, Dubeau F, Duncan J, Guerrini R, Kahane P, Mathern G, Najm I, Ozkara C, Raybaud C, Represa A, Roper SN, Salamon N, Schulze-Bonhage A, Tassi L, Vezzani A, Spreafico R (2011) The clinicopathologic spectrum of focal cortical dysplasias: a consensus classification proposed by an ad hoc Task Force of the ILAE Diagnostic Methods Commission. Epilepsia 52(1):158–174
13. Bote RP, Blázquez-Llorca L, Fernández-Gil MA, Alonso-Nanclares L, Muñoz A, De Felipe J (2008) Hippocampal sclerosis: histopathology substrate and magnetic resonance imaging. Semin Ultrasound CT MR 29(1):2–14

14. Bronen RA, Cheung G, Charles JT, Kim JH, Spencer DD, Spencer SS, Sze G, McCarthy G (1991) Imaging findings in hippocampal sclerosis: correlation with pathology. AJNR Am J Neuroradiol 12(5):933–940

15. Bronen RA, Anderson AW, Spencer DD (1994) Quantitative MR for epilepsy: a clinical and research tool? AJNR Am J Neuroradiol 15(6):1157–1160

16. Campos AR, Clusmann H, von Lehe M, Niehusmann P, Becker AJ, Schramm J, Urbach H (2009) Simple and complex dysembryoplastic neuroepithelial tumors (DNT) variants: clinical profile, MRI, and histopathology. Neuroradiology 51(7):433–443

17. Cataltepe O, Jallo GI (2010) Pediatric epilepsy surgery: preoperative assessment and surgical intervention, 1st edn. Thieme Medical Publishers, New York, pp 60–61

18. Cendes F, Cook MJ, Watson C, Andermann F, Fish DR, Shorvon SD, Bergin P, Free S, Dubeau F, Arnold DL (1995) Frequency and characteristics of dual pathology in patients with lesional epilepsy. Neurology 45(11):2058–2064

19. Cendes F, Li LM, Andermann F, Watson C, Fish DR, Shorvon SD, Dubeau F, Arnold DL (1999) Dual pathology and its clinical relevance. Adv Neurol 81:153–164

20. Chan S, Erickson JK, Yoon SS (1997) Limbic system abnormalities associated with mesial temporal sclerosis: a model of chronic cerebral changes due to seizures. Radiographics 17(5): 1095–1110

21. Cheon JE, Chang KH, Kim HD, Han MH, Hong SH, Seong SO, Kim IO, Lee SG, Hwang YS, Kim HJ (1998) MR of hippocampal sclerosis: comparison of qualitative and quantitative assessments. AJNR Am J Neuroradiol 19(3):465–468

22. Colliot O, Bernasconi N, Khalili N, Antel SB, Naessens V, Bernasconi A (2006) Individual voxel-based analysis of gray matter in focal cortical dysplasia. Neuroimage 29(1):162–171

23. Colombo N, Tassi L, Galli C, Citterio A, Lo Russo G, Scialfa G, Spreafico R (2003) Focal cortical dysplasias: MR imaging, histopathologic, and clinical correlations in surgically treated patients with epilepsy. AJNR Am J Neuroradiol 24(4):724–733

24. Cook MJ (1994) Mesial temporal sclerosis and volumetric investigations. Acta Neurol Scand Suppl 152:109–114, discussion 115

25. Crompton DE, Scheffer IE, Taylor I, Cook MJ, McKelvie PA, Vears DF, Lawrence KM, McMahon JM, Grinton BE, McIntosh AM, Berkovic SF (2010) Familial mesial temporal lobe epilepsy: a benign epilepsy syndrome showing complex inheritance. Brain 133(11):3221–3231

26. Davies KG, Hermann BP, Dohan FC Jr, Foley KT, Bush AJ, Wyler AR (1996) Relationship of hippocampal sclerosis to duration and age of onset of epilepsy, and childhood febrile seizures in temporal lobectomy patients. Epilepsy Res 24(2):119–126

27. Duchowny M, Jayakar P, Harvey AS, Resnick T, Alvarez L, Dean P, Levin B (1996) Language cortex representation: effects of developmental versus acquired pathology. Ann Neurol 40(1):31–38

28. Dumas de la Roque A, Oppenheim C, Chassoux F, Rodrigo S, Beuvon F, Daumas-Duport C, Devaux B, Meder JF (2005) Diffusion tensor imaging of partial intractable epilepsy. Eur Radiol 15(2):279–285

29. Dym RJ, Burns J, Freeman K, Lipton ML (2011) Is functional MR imaging assessment of hemispheric language dominance as good as the Wada test? A meta-analysis. Radiology 261:446–455

30. Fauser S, Bast T, Altenmüller DM, Schulte-Mönting J, Strobl K, Steinhoff BJ, Zentner J, Schulze-Bonhage A (2008) Factors influencing surgical outcome in patients with focal cortical dysplasia. J Neurol Neurosurg Psychiatry 79(1):103–105

31. Fernandez C, Girard N, Paz Paredes A, Bouvier-Labit C, Lena G, Figarella-Branger D (2003) The usefulness of MR imaging in the diagnosis of dysembryoplastic neuroepithelial tumor in children: a study of 14 cases. AJNR Am J Neuroradiol 24(5):829–834

32. Giannini C, Scheithauer BW, Burger PC, Brat DJ, Wollan PC, Lach B, O'Neill BP (1999) Pleomorphic xanthoastrocytoma: what do we really know about it? Cancer 85(9):2033–2045

33. Gross DW (2011) Diffusion tensor imaging in temporal lobe epilepsy. Epilepsia 52(Suppl 4): 32–34

34. Gotman J (2008) Epileptic networks studied with EEG-fMRI. Epilepsia 49(Suppl 3):42–51

35. Harkness W (2006) Temporal lobe resections. Childs Nerv Syst 22(8):936–944

36. Hedera P, Blair MA, Andermann E, Andermann F, D'Agostino D, Taylor KA, Chahine L, Pandolfo M, Bradford Y, Haines JL, Abou-Khalil B (2007) Familial mesial temporal lobe epilepsy maps to chromosome 4q13.2-q21.3. Neurology 68(24):2107–2112
37. Hirfanoglu T, Gupta A (2010) Tuberous sclerosis complex with a single brain lesion on MRI mimicking focal cortical dysplasia. Pediatr Neurol 42(5):343–347
38. Ho SS, Kuzniecky RI, Gilliam F, Faught E, Morawetz R (1998) Temporal lobe developmental malformations and epilepsy: dual pathology and bilateral hippocampal abnormalities. Neurology 50(3):748–754
39. Huang YC, Weng HH, Tsai YT, Huang YC, Hsiao MC, Wu CY, Lin YH, Hsu HL, Lee JD (2009) Periictal magnetic resonance imaging in status epilepticus. Epilepsy Res 86(1):72–81
40. Huppertz HJ, Kassubek J, Altenmüller DM, Breyer T, Fauser S (2008) Automatic curvilinear reformatting of three-dimensional MRI data of the cerebral cortex. Neuroimage 39(1):80–86
41. Im SH, Chung CK, Kim SK, Cho BK, Kim MK, Chi JG (2004) Pleomorphic xanthoastrocytoma: a developmental glioneuronal tumor with prominent glioproliferative changes. J Neurooncol 66(1–2):17–27
42. Katramados AM, Burdette D, Patel SC, Schultz LR, Gaddam S, Mitsias PD (2009) Periictal diffusion abnormalities of the thalamus in partial status epilepticus. Epilepsia 50(2):265–275
43. Keller SS, Mackay CE, Barrick TR, Wieshmann UC, Howard MA, Roberts N (2002) Voxel-based morphometric comparison of hippocampal and extrahippocampal abnormalities in patients with left and right hippocampal atrophy. Neuroimage 16(1):23–31
44. Keller SS, Roberts N (2008) Voxel-based morphometry of temporal lobe epilepsy: an introduction and review of the literature. Epilepsia 49(5):741–757
45. Kim DW, Lee SK, Chu K, Park KI, Lee SY, Lee CH, Chung CK, Choe G, Kim JY (2009) Predictors of surgical outcome and pathologic considerations in focal cortical dysplasia. Neurology 72(3):211–216
46. Koeller KK, Henry JM (2001) From the archives of the AFIP: superficial gliomas: radiologic-pathologic correlation. Armed Forces Institute of Pathology. Radiographics 21(6):1533–1556
47. Lach B, Duggal N, DaSilva VF, Benoit BG (1996) Association of pleomorphic xanthoastrocytoma with cortical dysplasia and neuronal tumors. A report of three cases. Cancer 78(12):2551–2563
48. Lerner JT, Salamon N, Hauptman JS, Velasco TR, Hemb M, Wu JY, Sankar R, Donald Shields W, Engel J Jr, Fried I, Cepeda C, Andre VM, Levine MS, Miyata H, Yong WH, Vinters HV, Mathern GW (2009) Assessment and surgical outcomes for mild type I and severe type II cortical dysplasia: a critical review and the UCLA experience. Epilepsia 50(6):1310–1335
49. Lin DD, Barker PB, Hatfield LA, Comi AM (2006) Dynamic MR perfusion and proton MR spectroscopic imaging in Sturge-Weber syndrome: correlation with neurological symptoms. J Magn Reson Imaging 24(2):274–281
50. Luyken C, Blümcke I, Fimmers R, Urbach H, Elger CE, Wiestler OD, Schramm J (2003) The spectrum of long-term epilepsy-associated tumors: long-term seizure and tumor outcome and neurosurgical aspects. Epilepsia 44(6):822–830
51. Madan N, Grant PE (2009) New directions in clinical imaging of cortical dysplasias. Epilepsia 50(9)
52. Margerison JH, Corsellis JA (1966) Epilepsy and the temporal lobes. A clinical, electroencephalographic, and neuropathological study of the brain in epilepsy, with particular reference to the temporal lobes. Brain 89:499–530
53. Meiners LC, van Gils A, Jansen GH, de Kort G, Witkamp TD, Ramos LM, Valk J, Debets RM, van Huffelen AC, van Veelen CW et al (1994) Temporal lobe epilepsy: the various MR appearances of histologically proven mesial temporal sclerosis. AJNR Am J Neuroradiol 15(8):1547–1555
54. Meiners LC, Witkamp TD, de Kort GA, van Huffelen AC, van der Graaf Y, Jansen GH, van der Grond J, van Veelen CW (1999) Relevance of temporal lobe white matter changes in hippocampal sclerosis. Magnetic resonance imaging and histology. Invest Radiol 34(1):38–45
55. Mittal S, Wu Z, Neelavalli J, Haacke EM (2009) Susceptibility-weighted imaging: technical aspects and clinical applications, part 2. AJNR Am J Neuroradiol 30(2):232–252
56. Oguz KK, Senturk S, Ozturk A, Anlar B, Topcu M, Cila A (2007) Impact of recent seizures on cerebral blood flow in patients with Sturge-Weber syndrome: study of 2 cases. J Child Neurol 22(5):617–620

57. Ozturk A, Oguz KK, Akalan N, Geyik PO, Cila A (2006) Evaluation of parenchymal changes at the operation site with early postoperative brain diffusion-weighted magnetic resonance imaging. Diagn Interv Radiol 12(3):115–120

58. Palmini A, Najm I, Avanzini G, Babb T, Guerrini R, Foldvary-Schaefer N, Jackson G, Lüders HO, Prayson R, Spreafico R, Vinters HV (2004) Terminology and classification of the cortical dysplasias. Neurology 62(6 Suppl 3):S2–S8

59. Parmar HA, Hawkins C, Ozelame R, Chuang S, Rutka J, Blaser S (2007) Fluid-attenuated inversion recovery ring sign as a marker of dysembryoplastic neuroepithelial tumors. J Comput Assist Tomogr 31(3):348–353

60. Provenzale JM, Ali U, Barboriak DP, Kallmes DF, Delong DM, McLendon RE (2000) Comparison of patient age with MR imaging features of gangliogliomas. AJR Am J Roentgenol 174(3):859–862

61. Sakuta R, Otsubo H, Nolan MA, Weiss SK, Hawkins C, Rutka JT, Chuang NA, Chuang SH, Snead OC (2005) Recurrent intractable seizures in children with cortical dysplasia adjacent to dysembryoplastic neuroepithelial tumor. J Child Neurol 20(4):377–384

62. Szabo K, Poepel A, Pohlmann-Eden B, Hirsch J, Back T, Sedlaczek O, Hennerici M, Gass A (2003) Use of preoperative functional neuroimaging to predict language deficits from epilepsy surgery. Neurology 60(11):1788–1792

63. Szabo K, Poepel A, Pohlmann-Eden B, Hirsch J, Back T, Sedlaczek O, Hennerici M, Gass A (2005) Diffusion-weighted and perfusion MRI demonstrates parenchymal changes in complex partial status epilepticus. Brain 128(Pt 6):1369–1376

64. Szaflarski JP, Holland SK, Jacola LM, Lindsell C, Privitera MD, Szaflarski M (2008) Comprehensive presurgical functional MRI language evaluation in adult patients with epilepsy. Epilepsy Behav 12(1):74–83

65. Taylor DC, Falconer MA, Bruton CJ, Corsellis JA (1971) Focal dysplasia of the cerebral cortex in epilepsy. J Neurol Neurosurg Psychiatry 34(4):369–387

66. Urbach H, Scheffler B, Heinrichsmeier T, von Oertzen J, Kral T, Wellmer J, Schramm J, Wiestler OD, Blümcke I (2002) Focal cortical dysplasia of Taylor's balloon cell type: a clinicopathological entity with characteristic neuroimaging and histopathological features, and favorable postsurgical outcome. Epilepsia 43(1):33–40

67. VanLandingham KE, Heinz ER, Cavazos JE, Lewis DV (1998) Magnetic resonance imaging evidence of hippocampal injury after prolonged focal febrile convulsions. Ann Neurol 43(4):413–426

68. Von Oertzen J, Urbach H, Jungbluth S, Kurthen M, Reuber M, Fernández G, Elger CE (2002) Standard magnetic resonance imaging is inadequate for patients with refractory focal epilepsy. J Neurol Neurosurg Psychiatry 73(6):643–647

69. Widjaja E, Zarei Mahmoodabadi S, Otsubo H, Snead OC, Holowka S, Bells S, Raybaud C (2009) Subcortical alterations in tissue microstructure adjacent to focal cortical dysplasia: detection at diffusion-tensor MR imaging by using magnetoencephalographic dipole cluster localization. Radiology 251(1):206–215

70. Woermann FG, Jokeit H, Luerding R, Freitag H, Schulz R, Guertler S, Okujava M, Wolf P, Tuxhorn I, Ebner A (2003) Language lateralization by Wada test and fMRI in 100 patients with epilepsy. Neurology 61(5):699–701

71. Wolf RL, Alsop DC, Levy-Reis I, Meyer PT, Maldjian JA, Gonzalez-Atavales J, French JA, Alavi A, Detre JA (2001) Detection of mesial temporal lobe hypoperfusion in patients with temporal lobe epilepsy by use of arterial spin labeled perfusion MR imaging. AJNR Am J Neuroradiol 22(7):1334–1341

Technical Standards

Pediatric Temporal Lobe Epilepsy Surgery: Resection Based on Etiology and Anatomical Location

Nejat Akalan and Burcak Bilginer

Contents

Abstract Advances in electrophysiological assessment with improved structural and functional neuroimaging have been very helpful in the use of surgery as a tool for drug-resistant epilepsy. Increasing interest in epilepsy surgery has had a major impact on adult patients; a refined evaluation process and new criteria for drug resistance combined with refined surgical techniques resulted in large surgical series in many centers. Pediatric surgery has lagged behind this evolution, possibly because of the diverse semiology and electrophysiology of pediatric epilepsy obscuring the focal nature of the seizures and frustrating the treatment of catastrophic epileptic syndromes specific to children. Unfortunately, refractory

N. Akalan, M.D., Ph.D. (✉) • B. Bilginer, M.D., MSc.
Faculty of Medicine, Department of Neurosurgery, Hacettepe University,
Sihhiye, Ankara 06100, Turkey
e-mail: nejata@tr.net; bilginer@hacettepe.edu.tr

N. Akalan, C. Di Rocco (eds.), *Pediatric Epilepsy Surgery*,
Advances and Technical Standards in Neurosurgery,
DOI 10.1007/978-3-7091-1360-8_4, © Springer-Verlag Wien 2012

epilepsy is more devastating in children than in adults as it interferes with all aspects of neural development. Nevertheless, during the last few decades, the efforts of a small number of centers with encouraging results in pediatric epilepsy surgery have motivated pediatric neurologists to gain interest. Although well behind in the number of patients compared with that of adults, pediatric series are increasing exponentially. While temporal lobe epilepsy is the focus of interest in adults, with almost 70 % of resections in the temporal lobe, the pediatric epilepsy spectrum is different. Resective or functional surgery techniques devoted to resistant extratemporal epilepsy are the major improvements in pediatric epilepsy surgery. Temporal lobe epilepsy in adults has been studied extensively but only recently has begun to receive attention in children. Several aspects of temporal lobe epilepsy in childhood remain unclear or controversial in terms of seizure semiology and its pathology. This is reflected in the surgical treatment. Information on the major contributors to a favorable outcome, such as type or extent of resection, in terms of seizure control and morbidity is not available as in adult temporal lobe epilepsy. This chapter discusses the major discrepancies between adult and pediatric temporal lobe epilepsy and outlines the current concepts in surgical treatment. The resection strategy based on the different substrates at different locations in the temporal lobe causing seizures is emphasized with respect to available literature.

Keywords Epilepsy surgery • Temporal lobe epilepsy • Temporal lobectomy • Children • Temporal resection

Introduction

The adult temporal lobe epilepsy syndrome (TLES) is well studied and understood by its clinical, electrophysiological, and radiological features. Offering surgical treatment is straightforward when drug resistance is a concern and the results of resective surgery in terms of seizure control are far superior to those of medical treatment [96]. In the adult epilepsy series, TLES is the most frequently encountered epilepsy syndrome as a candidate for surgical intervention. Mesial hippocampal sclerosis (MTS) is the most frequent surgical substrate, since it is responsible for more than 80 % of adult TLES. Temporal lobe surgery for intractable epilepsy is relatively rare in children compared to adults for several reasons. First, extratemporal catastrophic epilepsy syndromes associated with Lennox-Gastaut, Rasmussen's, and Sturge-Weber syndromes, hemimegalencephaly, and cortical dysplasia comprise a broad spectrum of the pediatric epilepsy surgery caseload. The incidence of mesial temporal epilepsy in children appears to be quite low in reported series, with only 19 documented cases among 2,319 patients with childhood-onset epilepsy, an incidence of 0.82 % [65]. While adult temporal lobe epilepsy in adults is most often manifested by partial seizures with autonomic symptoms, automatisms, and dystonic posturing, seizures originating from the temporal lobe have unusual semiology and electrophysiology, making straightforward localization in pediatric age patients difficult. In infancy and early childhood in particular, the auras are rare and difficult to recognize or are misinterpreted by family members. Automatisms, which are commonly seen in temporal lobe epilepsy in all age groups, are simple at a younger age and become more complex and discrete with age [29]; motor manifestations are usually symmetrical and tonic, clonic, or myoclonic in character, suggesting an extratemporal focus [74]. These motor manifestations, however, decrease with increasing age and are less abundant in adults. The severity of the condition varies at different stages of life, there is frequent interruption of follow-up in adolescence, and interpretation of the EEG is usually more difficult in children than it is in adults [37].

Surgical Planning in Temporal Lobe Epilepsy

The goal of surgery for drug-resistant epilepsy is to remove the hypothetical "epileptogenic zone" in the given cerebral area to eliminate seizures. The core of the epileptogenic zone is considered to be the pathological substrate described as an "epileptogenic lesion," which in most cases is apparent on imaging studies. In adults as well as in children, almost all temporal lobe epilepsy syndromes are related to a lesion that is visible with contemporary radiological tools. While MTS is the major pathological substrate in adults, mesial or neocortical tumor, dysplasia, or vascular lesion constitutes the "core" in children. Compared with standard neurosurgical intervention, the key point that makes the decision process different in epilepsy surgery is that the epileptogenic lesion and the epileptogenic zone do not necessarily share a spatial relationship. The epileptogenic zone may be within the boundaries of the lesion as in cases of dysplastic cortex, tumors of neuronal origin, and to an extent in MTS. Still, in the majority of TLES cases, the electrophysiological data related to the seizure activity extend far beyond the suspected lesion crossing over to relatively normal appearing brain tissue. For TLES, the major achievement has been the identification of the role of the mesial temporal region for seizure initiation in early 1950s [22, 27, 34, 35, 78]. The introduction of magnetic resonance (MR) has been the second major leap in surgical treatment because it allows the surgeon to see the anatomical substrate prior to pathological verification. Despite the fascinating advances in the diagnosis and treatment of drug-resistant epilepsy, the link between electrophysiological data and the anatomical substrate remains to be elucidated. Because of the inconsistent methods used for presurgical evaluation among centers, the different definitions of the epileptogenic zone result in variable recommendations for resection technique and extent. Even in adult MTS series, the most frequently encountered and well described focal epilepsy syndrome amenable to surgery, no single resection technique has been proven to be superior in terms of seizure outcome. When the lesion-dominated etiology of childhood temporal lobe epilepsy is taken into account, it becomes more difficult to define a stereotypical, standardized approach for a given case.

                                                                N. Akalan and B. Bilginer

Table 1 Distribution according to type of epilepsy surgery in adult and pediatric patients operated on between February 1996 and December 2009 at the Department of Neurosurgery, Hacettepe University Hospital

	Adult		Pediatric (<18 years)	
Surgery	No.	%	No.	%
Temporal resection	212	64.0	95	45.5
Extratemporal resection	106	32.0	52	24.9
VNS	6	1.8	12	5.7
C. Callosotomy	11	3.3	35	16.7
Hemispherotomy	8	2.4	23	11.0
Total[a]	331	100	209	100

All cases were operated on by the same group after being evaluated as drug-resistant epilepsy cases after first-line therapy, all with a minimum workup consisting high-resolution magnetic resonance imaging by a specific epilepsy imaging protocol, continuous video-EEG monitoring lasting 3–10 days, neuropsychiatric tests, and presurgical discussion at the weekly multidisciplinary epilepsy conference of the Hacettepe Epilepsy Group

[a]Some cases had more than one surgery of different modality

Table 2 Number of cases per type of surgery in pediatric TLES of different etiology

	MTS[a]	Tumor	Dysplasia	Nonlesional	
	No.	No.	No.	No.	Total
Temporal lobectomy[b]	27 (28.4 %)	16 (16.8 %)	5 (5.2 %)	16 (16.8 %)	64 (67.4 %)
Lesionectomy	–	8 (8.4 %)	3 (3.2 %)	–	11 (11.6 %)
Tailored temporal resection[c]	–	12 (12.6 %)	8 (9.5 %)	–	20 (21.0 %)
Total	27	36	16	16	95 (100 %)

[a]Mesial temporal sclerosis

[b]Temporal lobectomy refers to anterior 3–4.5 cm. Neocortical resection and mesial resection with amygdalohippocampectomy

[c]Tailored temporal resection comprises hippocampectomy and parahippocampal resection in all cases, with various amounts of mesial and neocortical tissue including the lesion

Patients

In this chapter, different approaches and their rationale are discussed based on the experience with 313 patients evaluated and operated on for drug-resistant TLES by the Epilepsy Group of Hacettepe University Hospitals, Ankara. Standardized adult and pediatric protocols and workup were used between 1994 and 2009 with a follow-up of at least 3 years (Table 1). Among the patients, 95 were under 16 years of age. The approaches for these 95 cases can be categorized as anterior temporal lobectomy (ATL), temporal lesionectomy, and tailored temporal resections (Table 2). The rationale for selecting the appropriate approach based on pre-operative investigation, the technique used, and the results are discussed separately for each group.

Presurgical Evaluation

The phase 1 study of children with a seizure disorder was performed primarily by pediatric epileptologists of the Hacettepe Epilepsy Group. The pool consisted of those who had already been evaluated by the pediatric neurology department and considered to be refractory to first-line medical therapy. After eliminating parent- or physician-related factors such as medication noncompliance and omissions and dosage errors, those who fulfilled the criteria of resistant epilepsy were accepted for further investigation. A routine EEG recording by a 32-channel EEG recording system, with the review of previous recordings, was followed by short-term EEG-video monitoring. MR images were obtained using either 1.5- or 3.0-T scanners (Symphony and Allegra, respectively, Siemens, Erlangen, Germany). The MR imaging protocol used for patients with epilepsy included coronal 3D T1-weighted (W) gradient-echo imaging (MPRAGE) obtained parallel to the brainstem, fluid-attenuated inversion recovery (FLAIR) images, and T2-W turbo spin-echo and T1-W inversion recovery images. Based on the preliminary data, if the referring epileptologist decided to expand the investigation, the child was hospitalized for continuous video monitoring at the EEG-video monitoring station until enough clinical and electrophysiological data were obtained indicating a focal seizure origin. Neuropsychological tests, essentially including measurements of verbal-nonverbal memory and attention (Wechsler Memory Test, Auditory Verbal Learning Test, the Stroop Test, and the Facial Recognition Test), were performed whenever the age and mental status of the child permitted. Those with enough evidence for a probable focal onset were discussed at the weekly conference of the epilepsy group, which comprised pediatric and adult epileptologists, neurosurgeons, a neuroradiologist, a neuropsychologist, and members from related disciplines such as nuclear medicine and neuropathology. The decision was made to either follow-up, perform further invasive and noninvasive studies, or perform surgery.

Of the 95 cases who had undergone temporal lobe surgery, 61 had a satisfactory neuropsychological test, 26 had an ictal SPECT, and 11 had a PET study in addition to basic evaluation prior to surgery. None of the cases in this select group needed a Wada test or invasive monitoring. The age of seizure onset for this group was 91.4 months (SD: 62.5) and the age at the time of surgery was 8.4 years (SD: 4.8). With the current protocol, the average period from initial admission to surgery was 8.3 months (SD: 3.8). The follow-up was done by the pediatric epileptologists every 6 months in the first 2 years to assess seizure outcome with the evaluation of psychiatric and social status. Standard follow-up protocol comprised a scalp EEG, MR study, and neuropsychological testing initially, tailored by the epileptologist in consequent controls.

Craniotomy for Temporal Approach

Regardless of the resection method chosen, almost all temporal lobe approaches were performed through a common frontotemporal craniotomy. The patient is

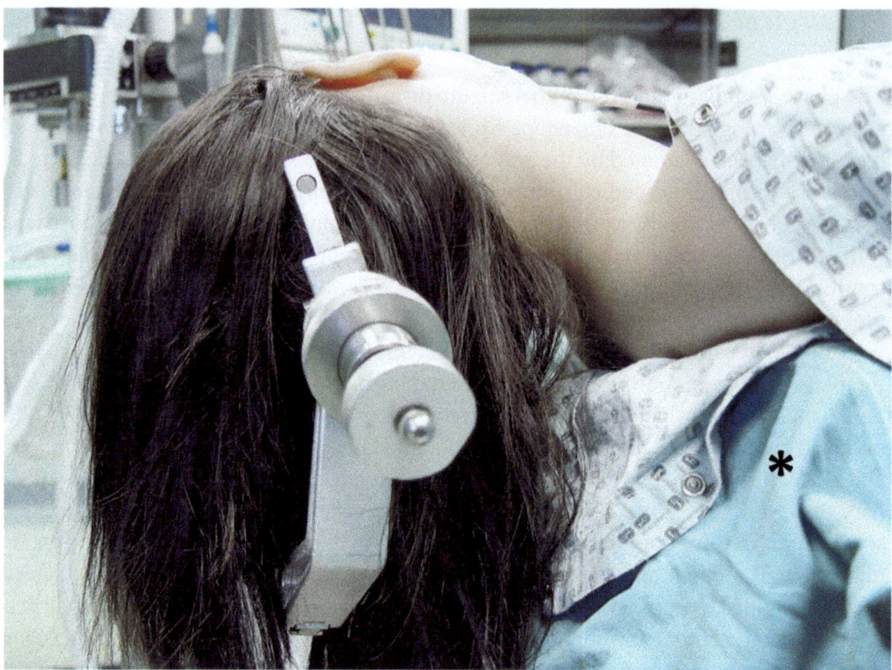

Fig. 1 The patient is placed in the supine position with the head turned to the contralateral side until the temporal lobe is aligned with the horizontal plane. The ipsilateral shoulder and torso should be elevated with a roll (*) to avoid traction to major veins and arteries of the cervical area

placed in the supine position with the head turned to the contralateral side until the temporal lobe is aligned to the horizontal plane. The ipsilateral shoulder and torso should be elevated with a roll to avoid traction on major veins and arteries of the cervical area (Fig. 1). Another option is to position the head and body in the lateral decubitus position. The axilla should be supported with a roll and a pillow should be placed between the knees to prevent nerve traction injury. A three-pin head fixation is preferred to accurately position the head unless the bone thickness is not available as in a very young patient. Horizontal head position with the head turned 90° to opposite side and parallel to floor provides a better spatial orientation for the surgeon, sufficient for superficial lesions. On the other hand, as most epilepsy cases require a thorough exploration and excision of the mesial-basal temporal lobe region, the position of the head needs further alignment for better exposure. The aim is to approach the base of the middle temporal fossa perpendicular to the horizontal plane and orientating the long axis of the temporal horn and hippocampus in a more vertical position. This can be achieved by readjusting the sagittal midline and axial axis of the head 20–30° to horizontal with slight neck extension so that the vertex points slightly to the floor, bringing the malar eminence to be the highest point (Fig. 2). The final position provides better exposure of the mesial-basal temporal lobe structures without significant retraction because the field of view of the surgical

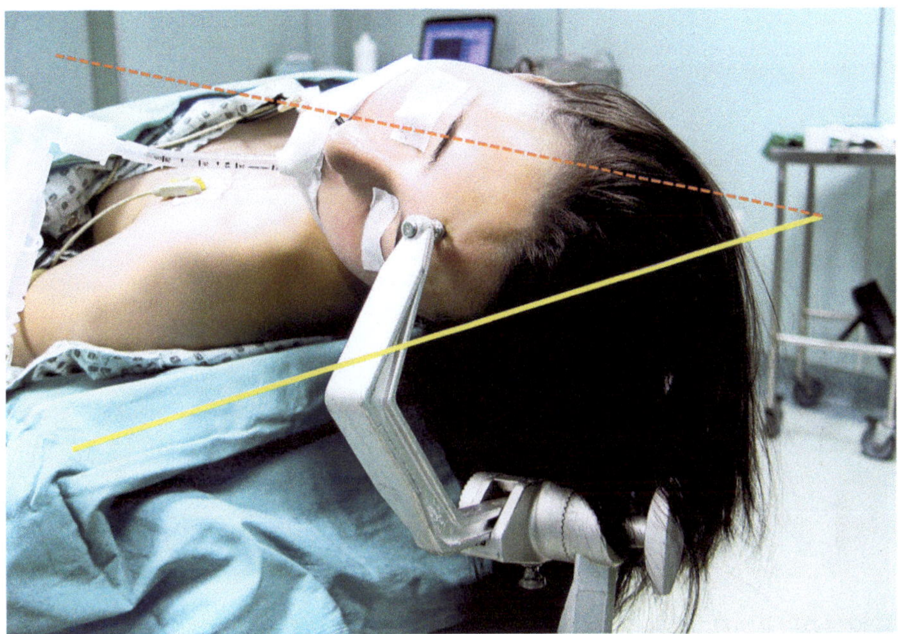

Fig. 2 Adjusting the sagittal midline and axial axis of the head (*red line*) 20–30° to horizontal (*yellow line*) with slight neck extension so that the vertex points slightly to floor, making the malar eminence the highest point. The aim is to approximate the base of the middle temporal fossa perpendicular to horizontal plane and orient the long axis of the temporal horn and hippocampus in a more vertical position

microscope is in alignment with the target. Similar to all other intracranial procedures in the supine position, the head and torso should be tilted up about 30° to ensure adequate venous drainage. Traditionally, a question mark incision that starts from the zygomatic arch in front of the tragus and extends above the auricle to the frontal hairline is preferred. Slight modifications concerning the size and the location of the skin incision and the bone flap might be required depending on the patient's age and selected target. Nevertheless, for resections aimed at the anterior temporal neocortex and mesial structures, a classical question mark skin incision, with the posterior curve over the superior aspect of the pinna and further anterior extension high above pterion, is not required at all. The skin incision, which starts at the tragus and with a smooth curve reaches the hairline just 1 cm above pterion level, is sufficient to visualize almost 6–8 cm of the temporal lobe from the temporal tip in a standard resection (Fig. 3). Temporal fascia, muscle, and periosteum are also sharply cut as a single flap parallel to the skin incision. Craniotomy, beginning with a key burr hole just behind the pterion, is kept as a 3-cm × 4-cm free bone flap without any additional bone removal from the sphenoid ridge or temporal fossa floor. These modifications provide a more comfortable postoperative period and avoid tissue swelling, future temporal muscle atrophy, injury to the frontal branch of the

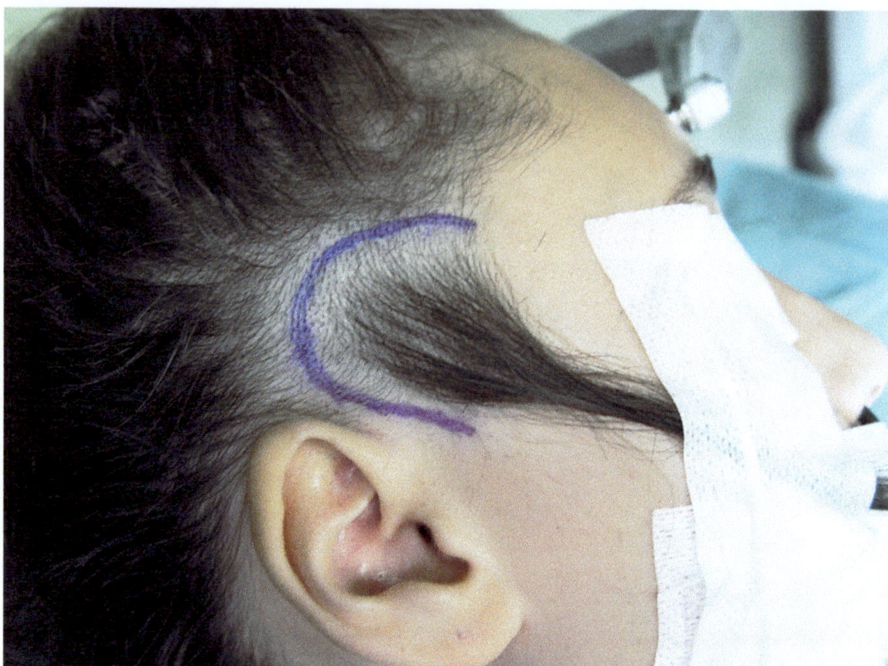

Fig. 3 The skin incision, which starts at the tragus and with a smooth curve reaches the hairline just 1 cm above pterion level, is sufficient for a standard procedure

facial nerve, and less epidural bleeding. A curvilinear or cruciate dural opening allows visualization of the sylvian fissure at the superior limit of the craniotomy, the superior and middle temporal gyri, and part of the inferior temporal gyrus inferiorly. The anterior border usually lies 2–3 cm behind the pole, while the posterior border allows access to 6–8 cm of the temporal lobe surface.

Anterior Temporal Lobectomy

Anterior temporal lobectomy (ATL) is the most frequently performed procedure for drug-resistant TLES. Except for neocortical lesions such as tumors, dysplasia, or vascular malformations, it has been the major procedure performed for clinically proven temporal lobe epilepsies. Although ATL is a widely used term, it does not totally represent the exact aim and extent of the procedure. This terminology proba- bly originates from the initial attempts at surgical therapy for temporal lobe epilepsy with the goal of removing temporal neocortical tissue as an epileptic focus. The role of mesial temporal structures was recognized in the late 1930s, and only after 1949 did Penfield and his associates extend the surgical resection to include the uncus and the hippocampus [18, 27, 33, 70, 71]. This strategy is further augmented by radiological evidence now provided by MRI that demonstrates the involvement of mesial structures in drug-resistant temporal lobe epilepsy, mainly in MTS. Currently, anterior neocortical temporal resection without electrophysiological and radiological evidence has been insufficient to relieve epilepsy [24]. Instead, removal of the mesial structures such as the amygdala, hippocampus, and parahippocampal gyrus is the target, accompanied by a variable amount of anterior temporal lobe resection, especially in "nonlesional" TLES. "Anteromesial temporal lobectomy" instead of ATL, which is originally described by Spencer, is a more appropriate term to describe the procedure, as proposed by Cataltepe and Weaver [18].

There is no consensus on a standardized approach for TLES with respect to the anatomical substrate and amount of resection. This is true even for adult MTS, the most frequently encountered and straightforward pathology in the surgical series. The discussion on resection limits in adult TLES focuses mainly on the assumption that the more epileptogenic area that is included in the resection, the more the chances for seizure freedom increase. Extended resection, on the other hand, is suspected to increase the risk of impairment in neuropsychological status, memory, and behavior [2, 25, 41, 47]. No solid data are evident, indicating a major advantage for either seizure relief or consequences among various modifications of mesial temporal resections with or without anterior temporal neocortex [25, 79]. Currently, anteromesial resections, including parts of the neocortex, are still widely used in adults, even in those with MTS.

Concepts Influencing Resection Strategy in Childhood MTS

There is no consensus on whether childhood MTS is an early form of the adult counterpart, where undiagnosed cases from childhood are eventually treated later in life. While MTS was the most frequent pathology in drug-resistant adult TLES, a significant proportion of those cases had a prolonged history of febrile seizures in infancy, almost three times higher than those without MTS [14, 19, 32]. Although initial data suggested a cause-and-effect relationship of prolonged febrile seizures and MTS, recent clinical and experimental evidence seems to contradict this hypothesis. Both experimental and human studies have not yet elucidated whether febrile seizures and MTS have a specific cause-and-effect relationship or constitute parallel processes with a common pathologic substrate [45]. Nevertheless, diversity concerning the etiology of childhood MTS is also reflected in several other aspects of the disease, including its prevalence, presentation, electrophysiology, and surgical strategy. The variation in MTS becomes more prominent when the child is younger, while MTS detected in adolescence tends to present in a more uniform fashion, resembling adult MTS. As mentioned earlier in this chapter, TLES itself is underdiagnosed, especially in early childhood, as reflected in a lower percentage of temporal lobe surgeries opposite to that in the adult population [9, 11, 12, 31, 37, 44, 75, 88, 90, 98]. Furthermore, MTS is not encountered often as the underlying pathological substrate in children. Overall, current data on childhood MTS is insufficient to define precise algorithms for designing a resection strategy [43, 64]. The current debate on adult MTS is mainly about restricting resection to the epileptogenic lesion present in the temporal mesial structures, i.e., selective resection versus standard lobectomy, which includes neocortical resection [6, 76, 79].

The concept of achieving equal success in seizure control with less neuropsychological impairment by performing limited resection does not seem to be valid for pediatric MTS for several reasons. While seizure control appears to be constant regardless of the resection type in adult TLES with or without MTS, data from experienced groups show conflicting results in children [43, 84, 86]. Although most of the contemporary series on pediatric TLES surgery reveal outcomes comparable to those of adults, the number of cases is far less than for adult series [43, 53, 61, 64, 86]. Comparisons are limited by the much smaller pediatric numbers because almost all pediatric cases with MTS had mesial resections combined with anterior lobe resection. One study from the Bonn group compared tailored surgery to standard resections [24]. Based on their experience with 89 cases of pediatric TLE, they have concluded that limited mesial resections based on electrophysiological and radiological data had less favorable outcomes compared to their experience with the adult series. While it is difficult to generalize this result based on a single study that had a limited number of cases, it may be the result of the clinical and electrophysiological peculiarities of childhood MTS or of nonlesional pediatric TLE. Therefore, with our current knowledge, the highly debatable statement that "the more epileptogenic area that is included in the resection, the more the chances for seizure freedom increase" seems to be valid for pediatric TLES. It is also more difficult to recognize and quantify morbidity related to mesial and neocortical resections, especially in young children. This stands as another important point against the quest for tailored surgery in childhood MTS.

Resection Strategy in Nonlesional TLES

The decision process in adults is debatable in those TLE cases without radiological abnormality. Patients with radiologically distinct abnormalities had significantly better seizure results than patients without obvious abnormalities [4, 59]. More recently, in selected subgroups of nonlesional or "cryptogenic" TLES, good outcomes comparable to those of MTS cases were reported based on interictal and ictal EEG findings and further investigation by SPECT, PET, and invasive recordings [26, 49, 83]. Nevertheless, no single investigation other than that of electrophysiology is capable of consistently differentiating a mesial or lateral focus to limit the extent of resection in nonlesional TLES in adults. In fact, a detailed seizure history combined with interictal and ictal findings alone is reported to provide enough information to differentiate the mesial versus the lateral temporal lobe source of seizures [13, 52, 72, 76, 93]. The pathological examinations obtained in nonlesional epilepsy cases rarely demonstrate changes that correlate with electrophysiological data. Nonlesional TLES cases or those with subtle MR changes constitute a higher proportion of the surgical candidates in children [6, 21, 59, 66, 85]. It is not yet clear whether this is due to the insensitivity of the current MR resolution to detect early changes of MTS under evolution or due to a distinct group not related to adult MTS at all. In children, it is more difficult to identify the extent of the epileptogenic region, especially to differentiate a mesial or a neocortical origin. Electrophysiological properties of the developing brain do not allow the epileptogenic zone to be defined as reliably as in adults [36, 44]. The variability of seizure patterns and the rapid spread of ictal discharges, especially in young children, make localizing seizure activity considerably more difficult [16]. Evidence from the current literature suggests that anteromesial temporal lobectomy is the treatment of choice for pediatric nonlesional TLE. Since 1996, the Hacettepe Epilepsy Group has used the Spencer-type resection in drug-resistant nonlesional TLES in children, no matter whether the preoperative workup suggested a mesial or a neocortical focus.

Technique

The combined removal of neocortical and mesial structures in childhood TLES is used almost uniformly with minor variations among centers. The variations include en-bloc resection of both anterior temporal neocortex and mesial structures, whereas a two-phase removal, as proposed by Spencer et al. [88], is most preferred as it is technically less demanding. The main modifications are related to the resection limits of both the neocortex and the mesial structure, mainly the hippocampus. In adult series, the posterior limit of an anterior lobectomy varies from 4 to 6 cm measured at the level of middle temporal gyrus, from the tip of the temporal pole depending on the dominance. In pediatric cases, this is approximately 3.5–4 cm, regardless of the dominant or nondominant temporal lobe. Sparing the superior temporal gyrus, especially that of the dominant hemisphere, is also recommended in adults because of concerns about language impairment [67]. A similar discussion about the extent of resection of the mesial structures with inconsistent results is possible. Because there are differences in presurgical evaluation, surgical techniques, and the assessment of the amount of resection in a large series from experienced centers, firm conclusions cannot be drawn from retrospective studies [1, 78, 94]. Nevertheless, pediatric TLE surgery can be regarded as in its infancy compared to adult TLE surgery; there are not enough data available on pediatric cases to discuss and speculate on variations of types and extent of resection in the temporal lobe. Therefore, each center has its own preference based on tradition and personal experience in pediatric cases rather than on scientific data. The technique described below is derived from the experience of the epilepsy team of Hacettepe University Hospital and has been uniformly performed in MTS and nonlesional TLE cases of both adults and children since 1994. Following exposure of the temporal lobe surface after craniotomy, as described earlier in this chapter, the intended posterior limit of the temporal neocortex resection, which is 3.5–4 cm depending on the age of the child, is marked on the middle temporal gyrus (Fig. 4). At this point the surgical microscope is brought in. The resection

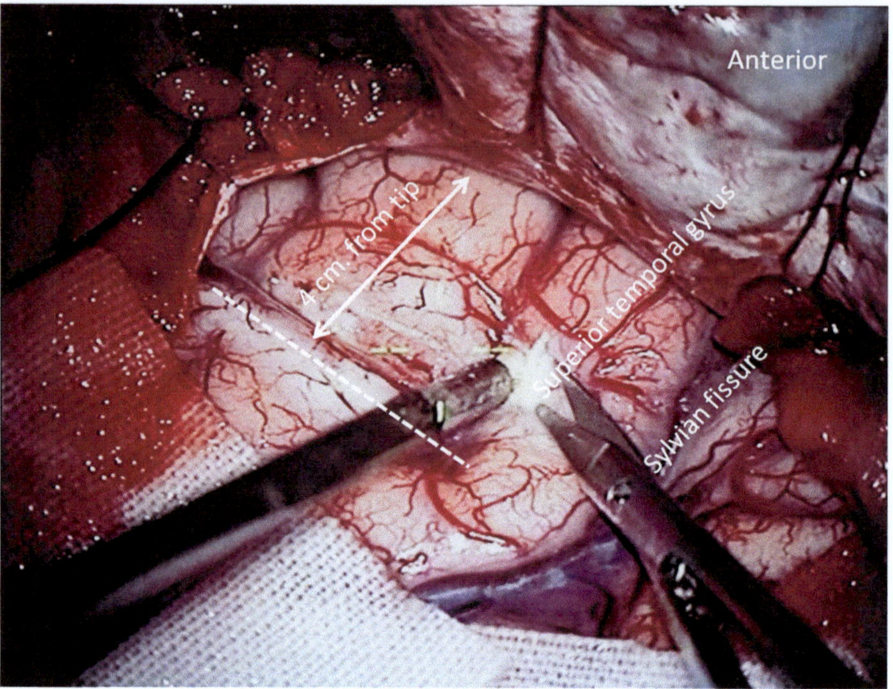

Fig. 4 Following exposure of the temporal lobe surface, the intended posterior limit of the temporal neocortex resection, which is 3.5–4 cm depending the age of the child, is marked on the middle temporal gyrus

is carried out with bipolar forceps and an aspirator, perpendicular to the long axis and toward the base and then parallel to the sylvian fissure, keeping the same depth within the white matter along the incision. Attention is paid not to enter the temporal horn at this stage. The most anterior part of the temporal horn over the head of the hippocampus lies about 3 cm from the pole, under the trajectory of the incision line. It is possible to recognize the ependymal border bulging within the white matter. Extending the incision to the pia facing the sylvian fissure is avoided at this stage. The incision line is sharply arched anteriorly in a direction parallel to that of the superior temporal gyrus, leaving 0.5–1 cm of cortical tissue between the incision line and the sylvian fissure to avoid unintended, premature opening of the pia facing the sylvian fissure (Fig. 5). In this way, no blood from the surgical area enters the sylvian fissure and vascular structures within the sylvian fissure are protected from traction and the effect of heat while working along the parallel axis at the mesial border. Both traction and heat effect on the middle cerebral artery branches may result with postoperative hemiparesis. It should be kept in mind that the sylvian fissure has a variable horizontal extension angle toward the temporal lobe that cannot be estimated from the cortical surface. Special attention should be paid not to enter the sylvian fissure while working on the superior temporal gyrus behind the sphenoid wing. This could

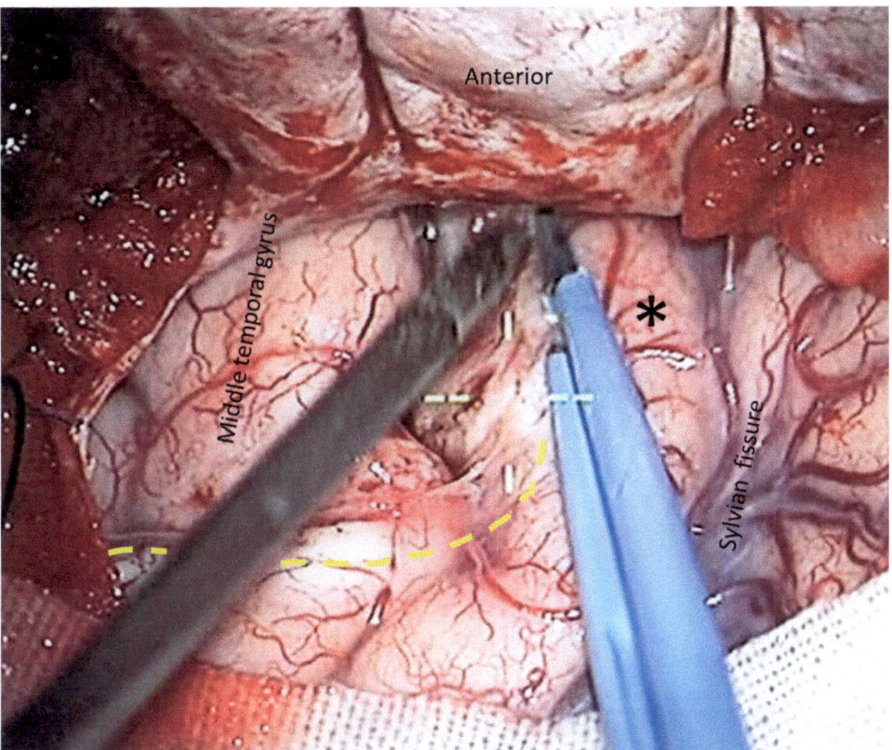

Fig. 5 Cortical incision starting at the 4-cm mark from the temporal tip (*yellow line*) is arched anterior to the superior temporal gyrus (*) , leaving 0.5–1 cm of cortical tissue between the incision line and the sylvian fissure to avoid unintended, premature opening of the pia facing the sylvian fissure

not only risk damaging the arteries and veins within the sylvian fissure but makes it difficult to perform mesial subpial resection at the later stage. Once the desired depth is reached in the white matter at the posterior and medial surfaces of the neocortical resection, the surgical microscope is aligned toward the base. The part of the cortical surface of inferior temporal gyrus that was beyond the craniotomy border in the beginning is now visible because of drainage of cerebral spine fluid (CSF) and aspirated cortical tissue at the incision line. The cortical incision is extended to the tentorium, with special attention paid to the vein of Labbé, which has a variable course over the inferior temporal gyrus, usually well behind the posterior border of the craniotomy. Patency should be checked at the beginning and just before the dural closure to avoid postoperative hematoma due to rupture. Once the lateral dura and tentorium interface is reached, the resection is continued subpially through the fusiform gyrus. Leaving the pia at the base intact avoids blood entering subarachnoid space and facilitates the removal of the mesial structures. Resection at the base is carried medially to the border of the fusiform and parahippocampal gyrus, which corresponds to the collateral sulcus. Subpial dissection is then carried out in an anterior direction at

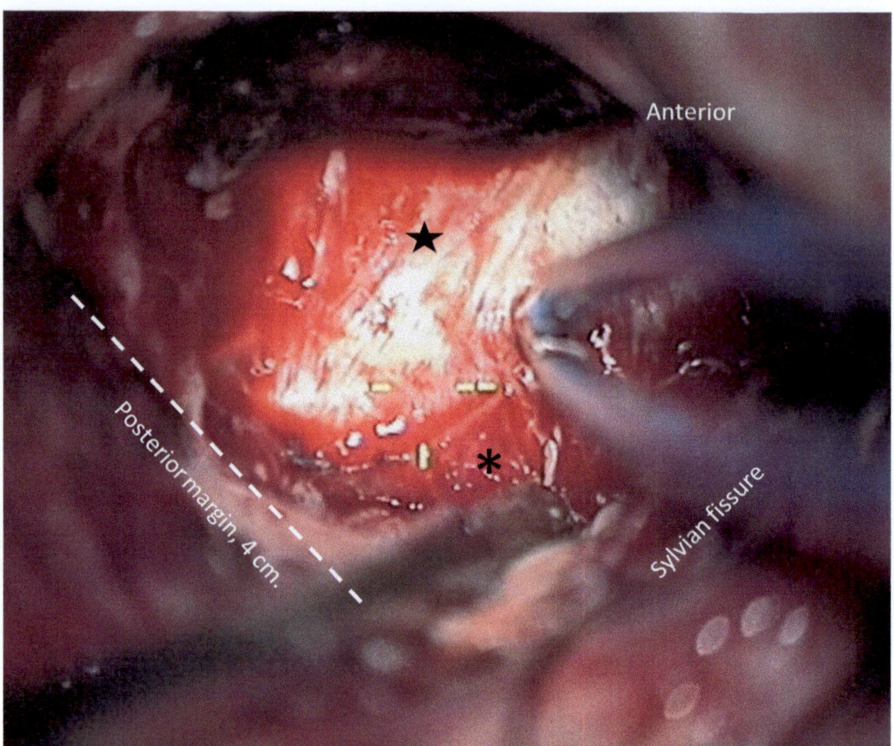

Fig. 6 The first phase of surgery is completed when the anterior neocortex is removed en bloc, leaving the pia (*) at the base to guide a safe mesial resection in the second stage. Dural base and tentorium are marked with a *black star*)

the lateral surface of the temporal lobe, working alternately from the posterior border and the anterior end of the incision at the superior temporal gyrus. Once both incisions are connected, the pia mater is coagulated and cut accordingly, releasing the anterolateral cortex. This completes the first phase of the operation to be followed by mesial resection and the remaining part of what is left from superior temporal lobe at the medial edge (Fig. 6).

The second stage starts with realigning the surgical microscope in the anteroposterior direction, facing the cut posterior surface, parallel to the long axis of the temporal lobe and mesial structures. The temporal horn is opened to visualize the head of the hippocampus. Unroofing the ventricle beyond the tip should be avoided not to damage Meyer's loop. The tip of the choroid plexus is visualized and secured by advancing a small cottonoid through the medial aspect of the temporal horn. A single 0.5-cm-wide self-retaining retractor is introduced to the roof, aligned to hold it and create enough workspace with microinstruments. With correct positioning and alignment of the microscope, the tail of the hippocampus can be reached without applying excess pressure on the retractor. The collateral eminence, head and body of the hippocampus, part of the amygdala with uncus, and the choroidal point

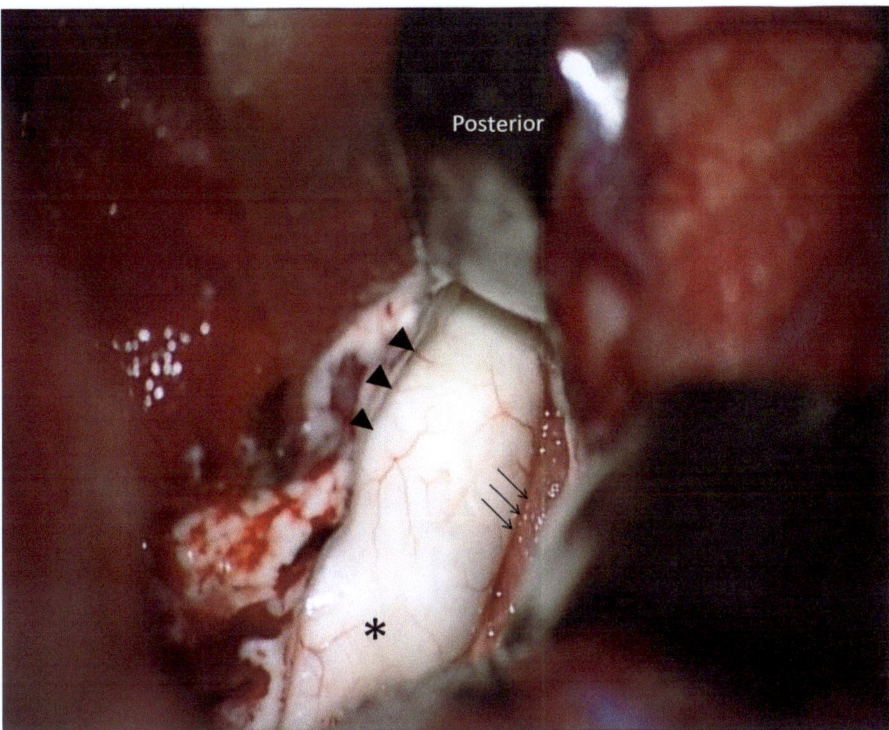

Fig. 7 Once the temporal horn is entered, a single self-retaining retractor is introduced to hold the roof to create enough workspace with micro instruments, and the choroid plexus is secured by advancing a small cottonoid through the medial aspect of the temporal horn (*small arrows*). With appropriate positioning and alignment of the microscope, the tail of the hippocampus can be reached without applying excess pressure on the retractor. Collateral sulcus (*arrowheads*), the head and body of the hippocampus (*asterisk*), part of amygdala with uncus, and choroidal point can readily be visualized

can be visualized easily. The rest of the operation can be carried out with this single retractor (Fig. 7). Resection of the mesial structures starts over the collateral sulcus within the ventricle that forms the lateral limit of resection. The groove between the lateral border of the hippocampus and the collateral eminence; the lateral ventricular sulcus is made deeper using a broad-based microdissector and aspirator until the pia is reached at the base. This incision is extended anteriorly outside the temporal horn between the fusiform and parahippocampal gyri through what is left of the neocortical excision. Posteriorly, the outer border of the hippocampus is followed, separating it from the collateral eminence and calcar avis until the tail is reached. Then the choroidal sulcus is visualized by holding the choroid plexus medially under a thin cottonoid. The fimbria is lifted up under high magnification, starting at the midpoint between the head and tail to expose the pial fold carrying the hippocampal veins and arteries. The fimbria is stripped a few millimeters while avoiding retraction or coagulation (Fig. 8). This is extended anteriorly up to the uncal

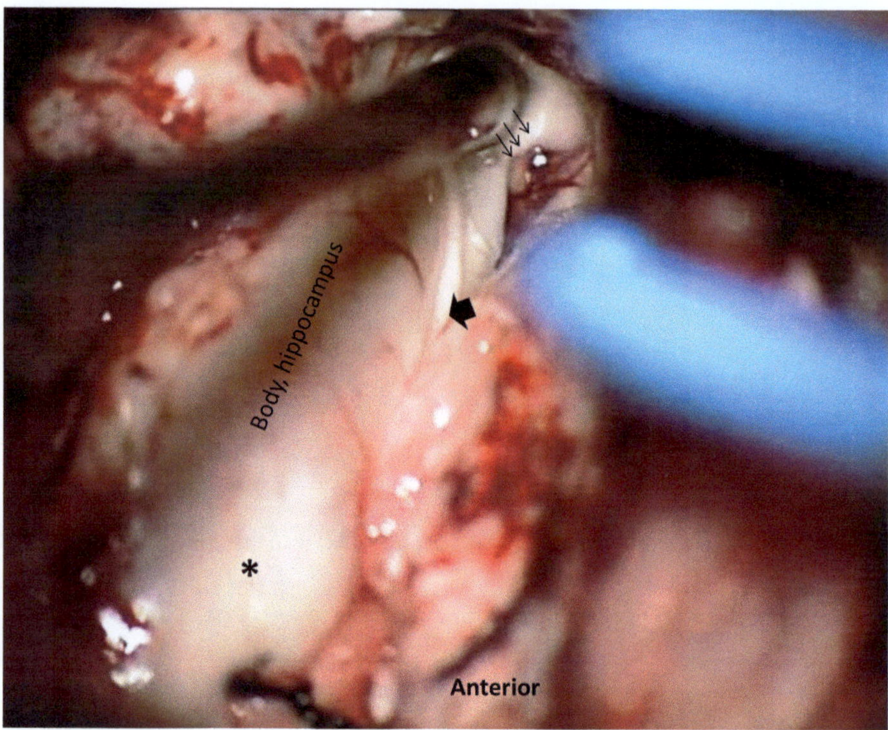

Fig. 8 The fimbria is lifted up (*small arrows*) under high magnification starting at the midpoint between the head (*asterisk*) and the tail to expose the pial fold carrying the hippocampal veins and arteries. A few millimeters are stripped from the fimbria (*arrow*) to avoid retraction or coagulation

recess to reach the velum terminale and posteriorly to the tail. Special care is given while dissecting the anterior of the choroidal point to separate the hippocampus head from the amygdala through the subiculum (Fig. 9). Separating the medial and lateral borders of the hippocampus from tail to head disconnects both the parahippocampal gyrus and the hippocampus, except at the far end of the tail and the pial fold below.

The next step is to carry the dissection around the head of the hippocampus to identify the most anterior part of the pial fold and the hippocampal arterioles within. The head is slightly elevated to expose the fold from the medial and lateral sides. With low-set micro-bipolar forceps, the fold is coagulated and cut in a stepwise fashion toward the tail while elevating hippocampal tissue. Once this fold and the corresponding parahippocampal tissue are cut, the whole complex with hippocampus and attached components of the parahippocampal gyrus can be removed en bloc after final dissection at the tail. At this point the microscope is aligned toward the temporal tip to start subpial stripping of the remaining superior temporal lobe remnants. Working from the anterosuperior aspect toward the base with the aspirator

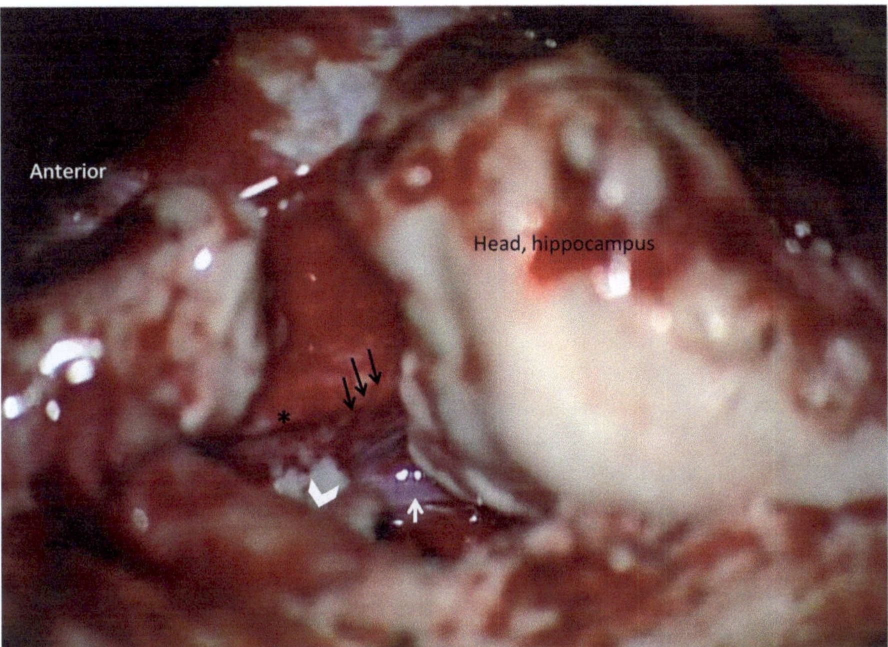

Fig. 9 Special care is given to the dissection of the anterior to the choroidal point to separate the hippocampus head from the amygdala (*arrowhead*) through the subiculum. Once the head is freed and elevated at the uncal recess, vascular supply is visualized at the pial fold (*arrows*) to be coagulated and cut. This is extended posteriorly to the tail (*asterisk*: free edge of tentorium under pia mater)

and dissector, the uncus and amygdala are reached without interrupting the underlying vasculature. The resection of amygdala must not go beyond the level of the MCA branches at the posterior-medial border to avoid entering the subthalamic region. Extensive traction or coagulation during subpial dissection at this area also carries the risk of damaging fine vessels from the MCA to the basal ganglia. This might be reason for some unexpected postoperative neurological impairment after an uneventful surgery. At the end of resection, the free margin of the tentorium, the third nerve, and posterior cerebral artery can be seen under the intact pia covering the crural and ambient cisterns. Following hemostasis, the corresponding layers are closed with an epidural drain under the bone flap.

Resection Strategy in Lesional Temporal Lobe Epilepsy

Among all the peculiarities of TLES in children compared to adults, one of the most striking features is the lesion-dependent nature of the seizures. Even in the more rarely encountered childhood MTS cases, chances for the existence of accompanying extrahippocampal pathology are much higher. The incidence of dual pathology in adult MTS cases is reported to vary between 15 and 30 %, while it was found to be up to 79 % in children and adolescents [10, 21, 28, 51, 57, 58, 64, 67]. In pediatric epilepsy surgery series, two thirds of cases are lesional cases, with tumors being the most common substrate followed by cortical dysplasias, nonspecific gliosis, and vascular malformations [50]. Tumors diagnosed as the substrate of drug-resistant TLES epilepsy have common and distinctive characteristics compared to other childhood supratentorial neoplasms [38, 48, 53, 82]. They are almost at the benign end of the pathological spectrum, mostly cortical, with a predilection for mesial localization, and show no symptoms or signs of neurological impairment except for intractable seizures [8, 17, 39, 79]. Dysembryoplastic neuroepithelial tumors (DNET) and gangliogliomas are the most common tumors encountered in most studies, followed by other low-grade gliomas and oligodendrogliomas to a lesser extent [48, 53, 82]. In our series, tumors constitute 38 % of all TLES cases under the age of 18 who were operated on, and half of the lesional cases (Table 2). None of the gangliogliomas (16 cases) were found at the lateral temporal lobe, while 8 of 20 DNETs extended beyond mesial structures into the lateral neocortex.

Malformations of cortical development are a common cause of developmental delay and epilepsy [3, 73]. They have been encountered more frequently with MR and consequently also in the surgical treatment of epilepsy in children. Although they tend to be extratemporal and multilobar in origin, they may occasionally present as TLES [20, 42]. Temporal lobe semiology is not infrequent either because of propagation from extratemporal cortical dysplasias or from those multilobar malformations extending partly to the temporal lobe. Focal cortical dysplasias restricted to the temporal lobe are frequently difficult to detect, and they are often disclosed only at pathological examination following assumed "nonlesional" lobectomies or as a dual pathology in pediatric MTS cases. A preoperative radiological diagnosis was possible in ten of our cases, including two tubers, while five others were detected only after pathological examination. If we take into account the various forms of lesions described as focal gliosis, abnormal neurons, or cortical derangement classified as "mild malformations of cortical development" in surgical material of MR-negative TLES cases, cortical malformations appear to be more frequent as a substrate. Studies on resected tissue and animal models suggest that abnormal neurons in focal malformations act as pacemakers for epileptic discharges, while epileptic activity in diffuse types is due to altered synaptic connectivity [53, 68, 80, 99]. Nevertheless, from a clinical point of view, the actual impact of developmental malformations, focal or diffuse, visible or not visible in MR, solitary or coexisting with another pathology, is not well established in childhood TLES.

Development of a resection strategy for a good outcome in lesion-related epilepsy surgery is far more challenging in children. Correlating the morphological and electrophysiological data and defining the borders of the epileptogenic zone that extends beyond the anatomical boundaries of a given lesion is more complicated in pediatric TLES than in adult cases. Presurgical evaluation in adults, including neuropsychological assessment, Wada test, invasive monitoring, and intraoperative electrocorticography (EcoG), that would allow definition of resection limits which would contribute to the outcome as well as the safety of resection is hardly possible

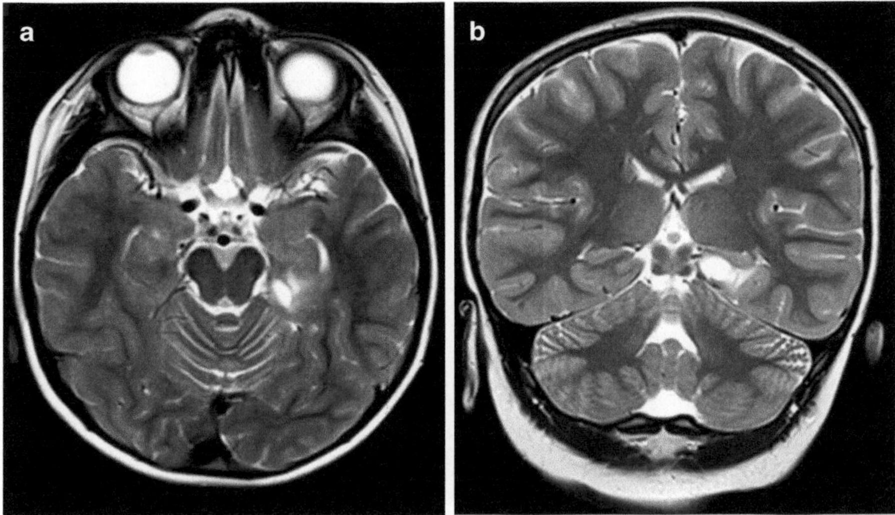

Fig. 10 Axial (**a**) and coronal (**b**) T2-weighted MR images of a DNET in a 4-year-old boy with drug-resistant epilepsy. The nonenhancing heterogeneous tumor is limited to the posterior parahippocampal gyrus and hippocampus, with no signs of invasion beyond the collateral sulcus to neocortex

in very young children. Moreover, the behavioral and structural plasticity of the developing brain and the impact of frequent seizure activity on neuropsychological function is highly diverse and makes it difficult to define a reliable preoperative baseline and to identify the possible risks of a planned resection [7].

Data for the decision-making process for lesional TLES in children are limited to reports from a limited number of series that usually were specific institutional experiences characterized by different populations of cases in terms of referral pattern, age groups, and evaluation algorithms. Using a broader perspective for resection strategy in drug-resistant epilepsy, it is practical to classify temporal lesions, regardless of their histological nature, into three major categories, discussed below.

Group 1: Lesions limited to mesial temporal structures (uncus, amygdala, parahippocampal gyrus, and hippocampus) with no signs of invasion beyond the collateral sulcus into the neocortex. Tumors such as gangliogliomas, DNETs, and occasionally low-grade astrocytomas represent the substrates for this localization (Fig. 10a, b). An abnormal appearance of the hippocampus due to developmental changes has been reported in association with agenesis of the corpus callosum, lissencephaly, and holoprosencephaly but rarely as a cause of resistant TLES [77].

Group 2: Lesions within the neocortex adjacent to mesial structures such as the superior temporal or fusiform gyrus and the temporal stem. Cavernomas, low-grade diffuse astrocytomas, and mild malformations of cortical development form this group (Fig. 11a–c).

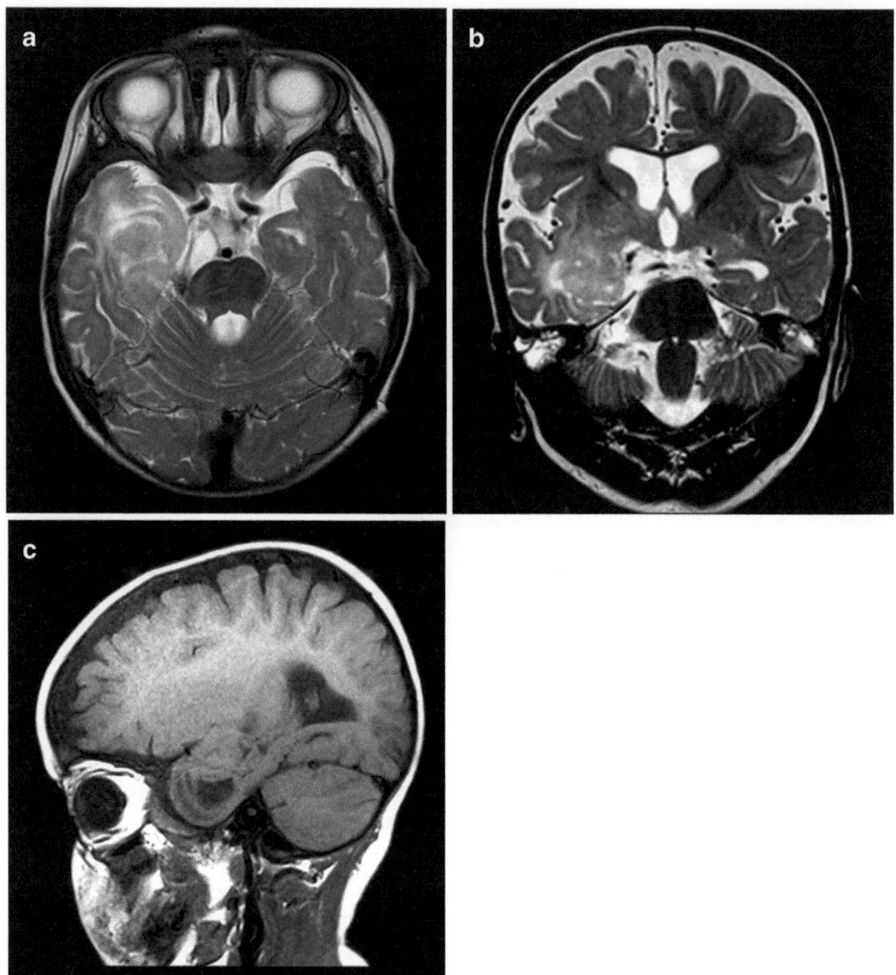

Fig. 11 Axial (**a**) and coronal (**b**) T2-weighted and sagittal (**c**) T1-weighted images of a glioneuronal tumor within the temporal basal neocortex adjacent to mesial structures. Invasion of the parahippocampal gyrus and hippocampus cannot be appreciated with in this current MR study

Group 3: Exclusively neocortical lesions, e.g., in the middle and inferior temporal gyrus and posterior fusiform gyrus at the level of the ventricular atrium. These could be DNETs, cavernomas, and cortical dysplasias of various types (Fig. 12a–c).

The resection strategy for lesions in group 1 is probably the most straightforward of the three. Resection limits of mesial structures in MTS or nonlesional TLES are more or less identical with the lesionectomy in this group. When there is clear radiological or intraoperative evidence for hippocampal invasion, a mesial resection utilizing the craniotomy and resection technique described above should

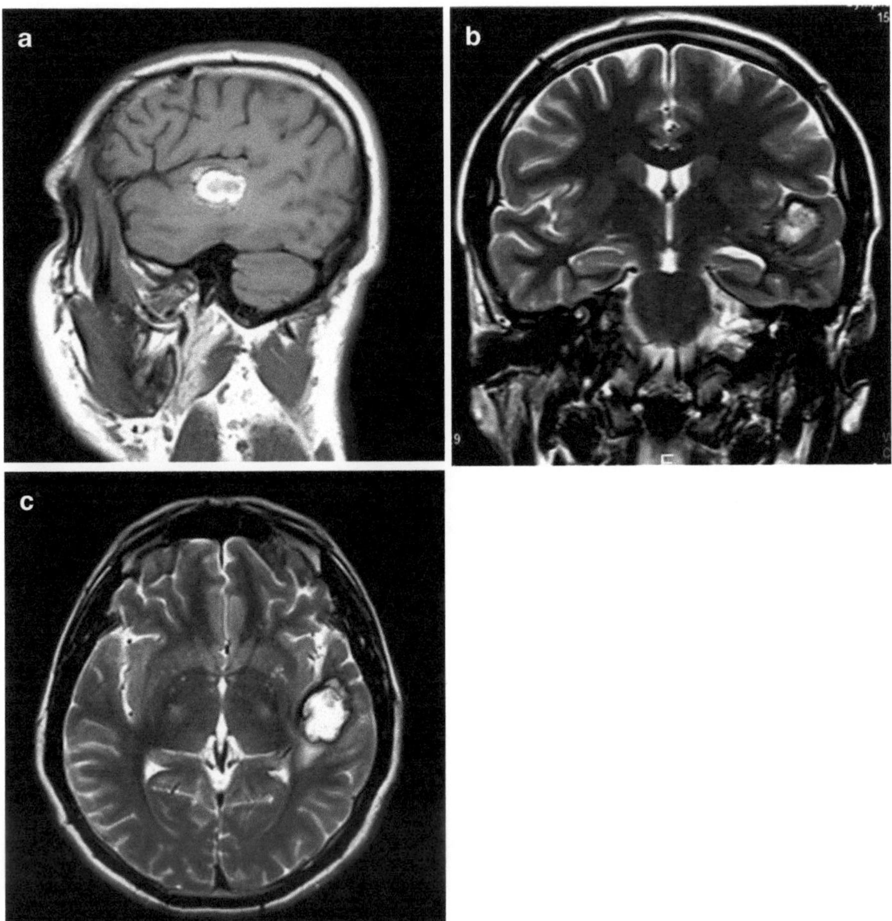

Fig. 12 Sagittal T1-weighted (**a**) and coronal (**b**) and axial (**c**) T2-weighted images demonstrating an exclusively neocortical lesion at the superior temporal gyrus showing a signal intensity consistent with cavernoma in a 8-year-old girl with drug-resistant epilepsy since the age of 2

be the treatment of choice. There has been discussion on whether to extend the resection into a temporal lobectomy. Based on the limited data from nonlesional TLES and MTS cases in children where tailored resections actually have less favorable results compared to standard lobectomies, we prefer to start with a limited anterior lobectomy followed by mesial resection of the lesion instead of transcortical lesionectomy. This tactic avoids unnecessary retraction of the overlying cortex or intrasylvian structures. Unlike in the selective lesional approach, normal anatomy and lesion limits are better visualized and a group comparable to nonlesional resections is obtained for further studies. Another topic of discussion is whether to include a hippocampectomy in those cases where the hippocampus is

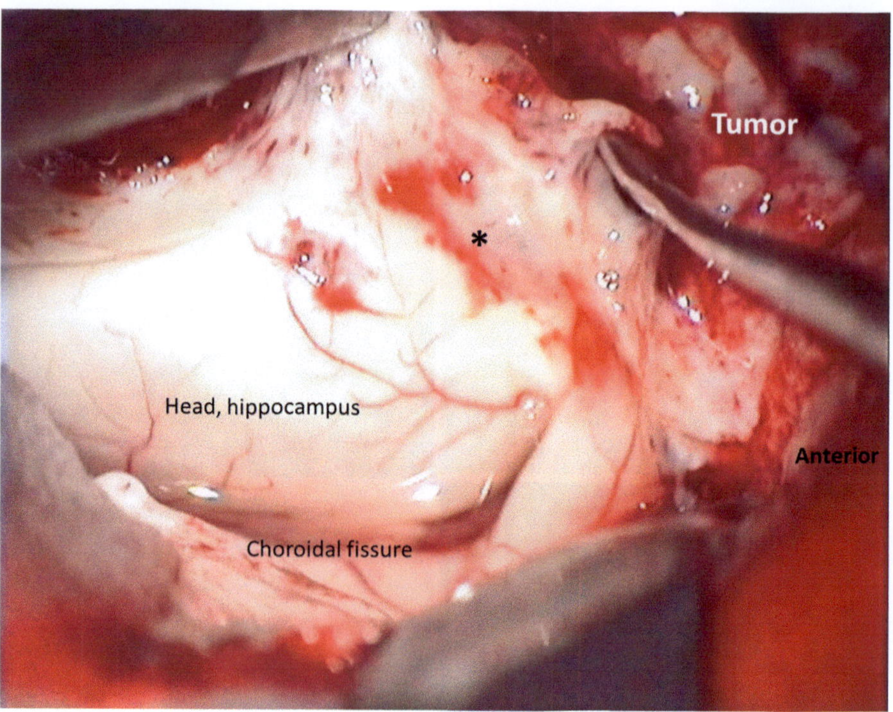

Fig. 13 Intraoperative view of the case through the temporal horn. Partial tumor invasion at the head of hippocampus and can be visualized over the ependymal surface (*asterisk*). This case also had a mesial resection, including hippocampus, in addition to the tumor

intact. It is generally accepted that the hippocampus is a very epileptogenic structure and may even act as a focus for secondary epileptogenesis. Until reliable radiological, clinical, and electrophysiological evidence is available to differentiate the contribution of the hippocampus to epileptogenesis in a given case, excision seems to be the best choice to achieve seizure freedom (Fig. 13). The same argument is more controversial in the approach to the lesions of group 2. There are conflicting results in the data from invasive recordings in primarily adult cases. Some suggest that the hippocampus can generate epileptogenic discharges without radiological abnormality when there is neocortical pathology, while others reported favorable results without including hippocampal resection [23, 56, 60, 95]. It is not possible to have this discussion in regard to the pediatric population since apart from the rarity of an exclusively pediatric series in the literature, it is not possible to apply a similar workup to children to obtain a logical answer. Currently, if the available data from electrophysiology and neuropsychological tests indicate mesial involvement, contrary to the MR study, we prefer to include mesial structures in the resection. Lesionectomy is preserved exclusively for cavernomas and for those who have demonstrated intact hippocampal function, especially on the dominant side in neuropsychological assessment.

Seizure is the most common manifestation of childhood supratentorial cavernomas, including those within the temporal lobe. They are believed to be highly epileptogenic due to the hemosiderin liberated from the oozing blood and easily detected by MR with their typical appearance. Currently, most of the cavernomas are detected as a cause of focal seizures well before irreversible secondary epileptogenic foci appear adjacent to the lesion. For this reason, lesionectomy for cavernomas should also include the hemosiderin rim within the normal tissue beyond the borders of the lesion. This statement can be applied to cavernomas in the temporal lobe within groups 2 and 3, justifying lesionectomy as the first line of surgical treatment.

Cortical lesions of the middle and inferior temporal gyri and the posterior temporal region of group 3 are good candidates for lesionectomy if electrophysiology demonstrates an obvious neocortical pattern without mesial involvement. Lesionectomy requires that special attention be paid to the adjacent cortex, unlike in excisions done for other purposes, because of oncological concerns. As mentioned earlier, except for certain types of cortical dysplasia and DNETs, which display abnormal neurons with intrinsic hyperexcitability, in most other cases the actual epileptogenic mechanism derives from the sum of morphological, biochemical, and excitability changes in the adjacent neural tissue. This might be considered preoperatively in MR to explain the perilesional hemosiderin deposits in cavernomas or adjacent dysplastic changes in DNETs, indicating a resection beyond the boundaries of the actual lesion. Unfortunately, in most of the remaining pathologies subject to excision, neither neuroradiology nor preoperative electrophysiology is sufficient for evaluating the adjacent cortex. Invasive monitoring is hampered by age concerns (although it is possible in older children) and any contribution of intraoperative EcoG is highly speculative in children as well as in adults because of its interictal character.

One other controversial issue is defining a strategy in "dual pathology" in which a cortical lesion accompanies an obvious mesial temporal pathology. When the accompanying cortical lesion is within the boundary of a standard temporal lobectomy or is close enough to be included by extending the excision without causing further morbidity, one may proceed with the resection. Otherwise, our strategy has been to target the mesial area first, leaving the lesion for further evaluation if the first step fails.

Complications

Currently, mortality related to an elective craniotomy for temporal lobe epilepsy in childhood should be regarded as extremely unusual; it is reported to be below 0.5 % in contemporary series, while morbidity related to surgery is between 2 and 8 % [13] In our series there was no mortality in the 95 cases of TLES. The most frequent complication is visual field loss, mostly as a homonymous upper quadrant defect, with an incidence varying between 9 and 22 % [5, 13, 54] In our series, eight children (8.4 %) were detected to have permanent quadrantanopsia at follow-up. This was due to mainly the compromise of Meyers' loop situated over the roof of the temporal horn, which is known to have a variable extension anteriorly. Extreme unroofing or retraction of the temporal horn during hippocampal resection is responsible for the majority of quadrantanopsia cases. Postoperative contralateral hemiplegia is the most serious complication of temporal lobe epilepsy surgery. It may be accompanied by language and verbal deficits when the injury is on the dominant side. Fortunately, this complication is quite rare, occurring in less than 1 % of the cases in contemporary series [43, 46]. Postoperative hemiparesis is attributed to several causes. Manipulation hemiparesis is believed to be caused by extreme retraction of the sylvian vessels which results in vasospasm or compression of MCA branches. Aggressive manipulation during resection at the mesial temporal lobe border without respecting the pial barrier is another probable cause of hemiparesis. This should be kept in mind especially when dealing with mesial tumors, where subpial dissection becomes challenging. A more straightforward injury pattern for hemiplegia is injury of the anterior choroidal artery (ACoA) branches. During amygdalohippocampectomy, vasospasm or occlusion of the ACoA due to traction or coagulation of hippocampal branches induces infarction at the posterior limb of the internal capsule. Two of our cases with mesial tumors had postoperative hemiplegia, but both improved almost completely within 3 months.

Neuropsychological impairment and psychiatric complications following temporal lobe resections are major concerns in adults [15, 78]. The current discussion on resection methods is considering outcome in terms of neuropsychological function more than in terms of seizure freedom. Reports from adult series that explore various aspects of postoperative memory functions indicate that almost one third of the patients exhibited a decline in verbal memory function when the dominant side is operated on [18, 69, 91]. Blume et al. [9] reported that psychiatric disorders occurred in 39 % of patients following temporal lobectomy for intractable epilepsy. Unfortunately, there have been few studies on neuropsychological morbidity in children after temporal lobe epilepsy surgery. Some studies found no major adverse effect of surgery on cognitive and behavioral function, while some demonstrated a minor decline only in verbal memory scores in some children in the early postoperative period [40, 81]. Only a few reports found that the chances for a neurocognitive decline are higher, mainly after dominant side resections in older children with high preoperative scores [30, 43]. On the other hand, improvement in intellectual function, behavior, and overall neurocognitive function following surgery has been suggested in several studies [40, 55, 81, 89]. The explanation for these inconsistent results in children compared to the adult population is probably multifactorial. Establishing and performing neurocognitive tests in different age groups is not as straightforward and objective as in adults. In addition, the neuropsychological features in childhood intractable temporal lobe epilepsy are not yet well defined and probably highly variable with respect to age and frequency, severity, and duration of the seizures. This makes it difficult to identify the actual preoperative neurocognitive impairment that would be subjected to change with resection. On the other hand, the plasticity of the immature nervous system provides greater capacity for functional reorganization in children and may explain the rather unaffected cognitive function regardless of the extent of surgery, unlike in adults.

Table 3 Outcome as Engel's classification based on 89 cases with regular follow-up not less than 24 months

Pathology	Outcome	Engel class I	IA	Engel class II	Engel class III
MTS [26]		19 (73.7 %)	18 (69.2 %)	3 (11.5 %)	2 (7.7 %)
Tumor [35]		33 (94.2 %)	29 (82.8 %)	1 (2.9 %)	2 (5.7 %)
Dysplasia [13]		7 (53.8 %)	7 (53.8 %)	–	4 (30.8 %)
Nonlesional [15]		8 (60 %)	7 (46.7 %)	3 (20 %)	3 (20 %)
Overall		67 (70.5 %)	61 (64.2 %)	7 (7.3 %)	11 (11.6 %)

Outcome in Pediatric TLES Surgery

Compared to adults, the temporal lobe in children is less often the major focus of intractable epilepsy. Recently, more interest in temporal lobe epilepsy and surgical therapy for intractable seizures has been generated compared to the more common extratemporal, partly catastrophic epilepsy syndromes of children. This is reflected in the lower proportion of temporal lobe surgery cases, unlike in the adult series. Information on the major contributors to a favorable seizure outcome, such as type or extent of resection, and morbidity is not as abundant as adult TLES. Surprisingly, reported children's surgical series demonstrate a high range of good outcome, similar and comparable to that of adult cases, regardless of the etiology, assessment methodology, or type of resection. Contemporary series that used comparable classification schemes, study populations, and presurgical evaluation demonstrated almost 80 % seizure control after surgery [13, 23, 53, 54, 62, 81, 82, 92, 97], Our results were similar: the overall seizure-free rate was 67.9 %, without differentiating for the pathological substrate. The breakdown of the cases demonstrated that this reaches 93 % when only tumors are taken into account (Table 3). On the other hand, there are also reports that long-term follow-up of temporal lobectomies in the young child shows a decline in seizure control over time [86, 87]. A lower proportion of seizure-free cases, down to 25 %, after 5 years has been reported in a limited number of cases [63]. Nevertheless, current data on the outcome of temporal lobe epilepsy in children seems to be very promising. These results are biased because of the relatively short follow-up time, heterogeneity of the pathological substrate, mixed samples (temporal and extratemporal, adult and pediatric), and relatively small number of patients in most of the series. Different referral patterns and definition of intractability and nonuniform preoperative workup among the reported series make it difficult to evaluate the overall outcome of multiple studies. At the moment these restraints preempt to discuss the ideal type and extent of resection for drug-resistant TLES in childhood.

References

1. Abosch A, Bernasconi N, Boling W, Jones-Gotman M, Poulin N, Dubeau F, Andermann F, Olivier A (2002) Factors predictive of suboptimal seizure control following selective amygdalo-hippocampectomy. J Neurosurg 97:1142–1151

2. Arruda F, Cendes F, Andermann F, Dubeau F, Villemure JG, Jones-Gotman M, Poulin N, Arnold DL, Olivier A (1996) Mesial atrophy and outcome after amygdalohippocampectomy or temporal lobe removal. Ann Neurol 40:446–450
3. Barkovich AJ, Kuzniecky RI, Jackson GD, Guerrini R, Dobyns WB (2005) A developmental and genetic classification for malformations of cortical development. Neurology 65(12):1873–1887
4. Bell ML, Rao S, So EL, Trenerry M, Kazemi N, Stead SM, Cascino G, Marsh R, Meyer FB, Watson RE, Giannini C, Worrell GA (2009) Epilepsy surgery outcomes in temporal lobe epilepsy with a normal MRI. Epilepsia 50(9):2053–2060
5. Benifla M, Otsubo H, Ochi A, Weiss SK, Donner EJ, Shroff M, Chuang S, Hawkins C, Drake JM, Elliott I, Smith ML, Snead OC 3rd, Rutka JT (2006) Temporal lobe surgery for intractable epilepsy in children: an analysis of outcomes in 126 children. Neurosurgery 59(6):1203–1213
6. Berkovic SF, McIntosh AM, Kalnins RM, Jackson GD, Fabinyi GCA, Brazenor GA, Bladin PF, Hopper JL (1995) Preoperative MRI predicts outcome of temporal lobectomy: an actuarial analysis. Neurology 45:1358–1363
7. Bernstein JH, Prather PA, Rey-Casserly C (1995) Neuropsychological assessment in preoperative and postoperative evaluation. Neurosurg Clin N Am 6(3):443–454
8. Bilginer B, Yalnizoglu D, Soylemezoglu F, Turanli G, Cila A, Topçu M, Akalan N (2009) Surgery for epilepsy in children with dysembryoplastic neuroepithelial tumor: clinical spectrum, seizure outcome, neuroradiology, and pathology. Childs Nerv Syst 25(4):485–491
9. Blume WT, Girvin JP, Mclachlan RS, Gilmore BE (1997) Effective temporal lobectomy in childhood without invasive EEG. Epilepsia 38:164–167
10. Bocti C, Robitaille Y, Diadori P, Lortie A, Mercier C, Bouthillier A, Carmant L (2003) The pathological basis of temporal lobe epilepsy in childhood. Neurology 60(2):191–195
11. Bourgeois BFD (1998) Temporal lobe epilepsy in infants and children. Brain Dev 20:135–141
12. Brockhaus A, Elger CE (1995) Complex partial seizures of temporal lobe origin in children of different age groups. Epilepsia 36:1173–1181
13. Burgerman RS, Sperling MR, French JA, Saykin AJ, O'Connor MJ (1995) Comparison of mesial versus neocortical onset temporal lobe seizures: neurodiagnostic findings and surgical outcome. Epilepsia 36:662–670
14. Camfield PR, Camfield CS, Gordon K, Dooley JM (1997) If a first antiepileptic drug fails to control a child's epilepsy, what are the chances of success with the next drug? J Pediatr 131:821–824
15. Cankurtaran ES, Ulug B, Saygi S, Tiryaki A, Akalan N (2005) Psychiatric morbidity, quality of life, and disability in mesial temporal lobe epilepsy patients before and after anterior temporal lobectomy. Epilepsy Behav 7:116–122
16. Cataltepe O, Jallo G (2010) Pediatric epilepsy surgery: introduction. In: Cataltepe O, Jallo GI (eds) Pediatric epilepsy surgery: preoperative assessment and surgical treatment. Thieme, New York
17. Cataltepe O, Turanli G, Yalnizoglu D, Topçu M, Akalan N (2005) Surgical management of temporal lobe tumor-related epilepsy in children. J Neurosurg 102(3 Suppl):280–287
18. Cataltepe O, Weaver J (2010) Anteromesial temporal lobectomy. In: Cataltepe O, Jallo GI (eds) Pediatric epilepsy surgery: preoperative assessment and surgical treatment. Thieme, New York
19. Cendes F (2004) Febrile seizures and mesial temporal sclerosis. Curr Opin Neurol 17:161–164
20. Cepeda C, André VM, Flores-Hernández J, Nguyen OK, Wu N, Klapstein GJ, Nguyen S, Koh S, Vinters HV, Levine MS, Mathern GW (2005) Pediatric cortical dysplasia: correlations between neuroimaging, electrophysiology and location of cytomegalic neurons and balloon cells and glutamate/GABA synaptic circuits. Dev Neurosci 27(1):59–76
21. Cervenka MC, Hartman AL (2010) Mesial temporal sclerosis in children. In: Cataltepe O, Jallo GI (eds) Pediatric epilepsy surgery: preoperative assessment and surgical treatment. Thieme, New York
22. Clusmann H (2008) Predictors, procedures, and perspective for temporal lobe epilepsy surgery. Semin Ultrasound CT MR 29(1):60–70

23. Clusmann H, Kral T, Fackeldey E, Blümcke I, Helmstaedter C, von Oertzen J, Urbach H, Schramm J (2004) Lesional mesial temporal lobe epilepsy and limited resections: prognostic factors and outcome. J Neurol Neurosurg Psychiatry 75(11):1589–1596
24. Clusmann H, Kral T, Gleissner U, Sassen R, Urbach H, Blumcke I, Bogucki J, Schramm J (2004) Analysis of different types of resection for pediatric patients with temporal lobe epilepsy. Neurosurgery 54:847–859
25. Clusmann H, Schramm J, Kral T, Helmstaedter C, Ostertun B, Fimmers R, Haun D, Elger CE (2002) Prognostic factors and outcome after different types of resection for temporal lobe epilepsy. J Neurosurg 97:1131–1141
26. Cukiert A, Burattini JA, Mariani PP, Cukiert CM, Argentoni M, Baise-Zung C, Forster CR, Mello VA (2010) Outcome after cortico-amygdalo-hippocampectomy in patients with temporal lobe epilepsy and normal MRI. Seizure 19(6):319–323
27. de Almeida AN, Teixeira MJ, Feindel WH (2008) From lateral to mesial: the quest for a surgical cure for temporal lobe epilepsy. Epilepsia 49:98–107
28. Dericioglu N, Oguz KK, Soylemezoglu F, Akalan N, Saygi S (2009) Resective surgery is possible in patients with temporal lobe epilepsy due to bilateral isolated hippocampal malformation. Clin Neurol Neurosurg 6:554–557
29. Dlugos DJ (2001) The early identification of candidates for epilepsy surgery. Arch Neurol 58(10):1543–1546
30. Dlugos DJ, Moss EM, Duhaime AC, Brooks-Kayal AR (1999) Language-related cognitive declines after left temporal lobectomy in children. Pediatr Neurol 21(1):444–449
31. Duchowny M, Levin B, Jayakar P, Resnick T, Alvarez L, Morrison G, Dean P (1992) Temporal lobectomy in early childhood. Epilepsia 33(2):298–303
32. Falconer MA, Serafetinides EA, Corselis JAN (1964) Etiology and pathogenesis of temporal lobe epilepsy. Arch Neurol 10:233–248
33. Falconer MA (1953) Discussion on the surgery of temporal lobe epilepsy: surgical and pathological results. Proc R Soc Med 46:971–974
34. Feindel W, Penfield W (1954) Localization of discharge in temporal lobe automatism. Arch Neurol Psychiatry 72:605–630
35. Feindel W, Penfield W, Jasper H (1952) Localization of epileptic discharge in temporal lobe automatism. Trans Am Neurol Assoc 77:14–17
36. Fogarasi A, Tuxhorn I, Janszky J, Janszky I, Rásonyi G, Kelemen A, Halász P (2007) Age-dependent seizure semiology in temporal lobe epilepsy. Epilepsia 48(9):1697–1702
37. Franzon RC, Montenegro MA, Guimarães CA, Guerreiro CA, Cendes F, Guerreiro MM (2004) Clinical, electroencephalographic, and behavioral features of temporal lobe epilepsy in childhood. J Child Neurol 19(6):418–423
38. Fried I, Kim JH, Spencer DD (1994) Limbic and neocortical gliomas associated with intractable seizures: a distinct clinicopathological group. Neurosurgery 34(5):815–823
39. Giulioni M, Galassi E, Zucchelli M, Volpi L (2005) Seizure outcome of lesionectomy in glioneuronal tumors associated with epilepsy in children. J Neurosurg 102(3 Suppl):288–293
40. Gleissner U, Sassen R, Lendt M, Clusmann H, Elger CE, Helmstaedter C (2002) Pre- and postoperative verbal memory in pediatric patients with temporal lobe epilepsy. Epilepsy Res 51:287–296
41. Goldstein LH, Polkey CE (1993) Short-term cognitive changes after unilateral temporal lobectomy or unilateral amygdalo-hippocampectomy for the relief of temporal lobe epilepsy. J Neurol Neurosurg Psychiatry 56:135–140
42. Hamiwka LD, Grondin RT, Madsen JR (2010) Surgical approaches in cortical dysplasia. In: Cataltepe O, Jallo GI (eds) Pediatric epilepsy surgery: preoperative assessment and surgical treatment. Thieme, New York
43. Harkness W (2006) Temporal lobe resections. Childs Nerv Syst 22:936–944
44. Harvey AS, Berkovic SF, Wrennall JA, Hopkins IJ (1997) Temporal lobe epilepsy in childhood: clinical, EEG, and neuroimaging findings and syndrome classification in a cohort with new-onset seizures. Neurology 49:960–968

45. Haut SR, Moshe SL (2006) Is mesial temporal sclerosis caused by early childhood neurological insults? In: Miller JV, Silbergeld DL (eds) Epilepsy surgery: principles and controversies. Taylor & Francis, New York/London

46. Helgason CM, Bergen D, Bleck TP, Morrell F, Whisler WW (1987) Infarction after surgery for focal epilepsy. Epilepsia 28:340–345

47. Helmstaedter C, Elger CE, Hufnagel A, Zentner J, Schramm J (1996) Different effects of left anterior temporal lobectomy, selective amygdalohippocampectomy, and temporal cortical lesionectomy on verbal learning, memory, and recognition. J Epilepsy 9:39–45

48. Hennessy MJ, Elwes RD, Honavar M, Rabe-Hesketh S, Binnie CD, Polkey CE (2001) Predictors of outcome and pathological considerations in the surgical treatment of intractable epilepsy associated with temporal lobe lesions. J Neurol Neurosurg Psychiatry 70(4):450–458

49. Holmes MD, Born DE, Kutsy RL, Wilensky AJ, Ojemann GA, Ojemann LM (2000) Outcome after surgery in patients with refractory temporal lobe epilepsy and normal MRI. Seizure 9:407–411

50. Ianelli A, Guzetta F, Battaglia D, Iuvone L, Di Rocco C (2000) Surgical treatment of temporal tumors associated with epilepsy in children. Pediatr Neurosurg 32:248–254

51. Jay V, Becker LE, Otsubo H, Hwang PA, Hoffman HJ, Harwood-Nash D (1993) Pathology of temporal lobectomy for refractory seizures in children. J Neurosurg 79:53–61

52. Jung WY, Pacia SV, Devinsky R (1999) Neocortical temporal lobe epilepsy: intracranial EEG features and surgical outcome. J Clin Neurophysiol 16:419–425

53. Kan P, Van Orman C, Kestle JR (2008) Outcomes after surgery for focal epilepsy in children. Childs Nerv Syst 24(5):587–591

54. Karatas H, Gurer G, Pinar A, Soylemezoglu F, Tezel GG, Hascelik G, Akalan N, Tuncer S, Ciger A, Saygi S (2008) Investigation of HSV-1, HSV-2, CMV, HHV-6 and HHV-8 DNA by real-time PCR in surgical resection materials of epilepsy patients with mesial temporal lobe sclerosis. J Neurol Sci 264(1–2):151–156

55. Kim SK, Wang KC, Hwang YS, Kim KJ, Chae JH, Kim IO, Cho BK (2008) Epilepsy surgery in children: outcomes and complications. J Neurosurg Pediatr 1(4):277–283

56. Lah S (2008) Neuropsychological assessment in epilepsy surgery of children. Neurochirurgie 54(3):245–252

57. Lee SK, Lee SY, Kim KK, Hong KS, Lee DS, Chung CK (2005) Surgical outcome and prognostic factors of cryptogenic neocortical epilepsy. Ann Neurol 58(4):525–532

58. Lévesque MF, Nakasato N, Vinters HV, Babb TL (1991) Surgical treatment of limbic epilepsy associated with extrahippocampal lesions: the problem of dual pathology. J Neurosurg 75(3):364–370

59. Li LM, Cendes F, Watson C, Andermann F, Fish DR, Dubeau F, Free S, Olivier A, Harkness W, Thomas DG, Duncan JS, Sander JW, Shorvon SD, Cook MJ, Arnold DL (1997) Surgical treatment of patients with single and dual pathology: relevance of lesion and of hippocampal atrophy to seizure outcome. Neurology 48(2):437–444

60. LoPinto-Khoury C, Sperling MR, Skidmore C, Nei M, Evans J, Sharan A, Mintzer S (2012) Surgical outcome in PET-positive, MRI-negative patients with temporal lobe epilepsy. Epilepsia 53(2):342–348

61. Mathern GW, Babb TL, Pretorius JK, Melendez M, Lévesque MF (1995) The pathophysiologic relationships between lesion pathology, intracranial ictal EEG onsets, and hippocampal neuron losses in temporal lobe epilepsy. Epilepsy Res 21(2):133–147

62. Maton B, Jayakar P, Resnick T, Morrison G, Ragheb J, Duchowny M (2008) Surgery for medically intractable temporal lobe epilepsy during early life. Epilepsia 49(1):80–87

63. McIntosh AM, Wilson SJ, Berkovic SF (2001) Seizure outcome after temporal lobectomy: current research practice and findings. Epilepsia 42:1288–1307

64. Mizrahi EM, Kellaway P, Grossman RG et al (1990) Anterior temporal lobectomy and medically refractory temporal lobe epilepsy of childhood. Epilepsia 31:302–312

65. Mohamed A, Wyllie E, Ruggieri P, Kotagal P, Babb T, Hilbig A, Wylie C, Ying Z, Staugaitis S, Najm I, Bulacio J, Foldvary N, Lüders H, Bingaman W (2001) Temporal lobe epilepsy due

to hippocampal sclerosis in pediatric candidates for epilepsy surgery. Neurology 56(12):1643–1649

66. Murakami N, Ohno S, Oka E, Tanaka A (1996) Mesial temporal lobe epilepsy in childhood. Epilepsia 37(suppl 3):52–56

67. Ng YT, McGregor AL, Duane DC, Jahnke HK, Bird CR, Wheless JW (2006) Childhood mesial temporal sclerosis. J Child Neurol 21(6):512–517

68. Ojemann JG (2010) Tailored temporal lobectomy techniques. In: Cataltepe O, Jallo GI (eds) Stuttgart pediatric epilepsy surgery: preoperative assesment and surgical treatment. Thieme, New York

69. Ozbas-Gerçeker F, Redeker S, Boer K, Ozgüç M, Saygi S, Dalkara T, Soylemezoglu F, Akalan N, Baayen JC, Gorter JA, Aronica E (2006) Serial analysis of gene expression in the hippocampus of patients with mesial temporal lobe epilepsy. Neuroscience 138(2):457–474

70. Paglioli E, Palmini A, Portuguez M, Paglioli E, Azambuja N, da Costa JC, da Silva Filho HF, Martinez JV, Hoeffel JR (2006) Seizure and memory outcome following temporal lobe surgery: selective compared with nonselective approaches for hippocampal sclerosis. J Neurosurg 104(1):70–78

71. Penfield W, Flanigin H (1950) Surgical therapy of temporal lobe seizures. AMA Arch Neurol Psychiatry 64(4):491–500

72. Penfield W, Flanigin H (1952) Temporal lobe seizures and the technique of subtemporal lobectomy. Ann Surg 134:625–634

73. Pfänder M, Arnold S, Henkel A, Weil S, Werhahn KJ, Eisensehr I, Winkler PA, Noachtar S (2002) Clinical features and EEG findings differentiating mesial from neocortical temporal lobe epilepsy. Epileptic Disord 4:189–195

74. Porter BE, Judkins AR, Clancy RR, Duhaime A, Dlugos DJ, Golden JA (2003) Dysplasia: a common finding in intractable pediatric temporal lobe epilepsy. Neurology 61(3):365–368

75. Ray A, Kotagal P (2005) Temporal lobe epilepsy in children: overview of clinical semiology. Epileptic Disord 7(4):299–307

76. Rye A, Wyllie E (2005) Treatment options and paradigms in childhood temporal lobe epilepsy. Expert Rev Neurother 5(6):785–801

77. Sagher O, Thawani JP, Etame AB, Gomez-Hassan DM (2012) Seizure outcomes and mesial resection volumes following selective amygdalohippocampectomy and temporal lobectomy. Neurosurg Focus 32(3):E8

78. Sato N, Hatakeyama S, Shimizu N, Hikima A, Aoki J, Endo K (2001) MR evaluation of the hippocampus in patients with congenital malformations of the brain. AJNR Am J Neuroradiol 22(2):389–393

79. Schramm J (2008) Temporal lobe epilepsy surgery and the quest for optimal extent of resection: a review. Epilepsia 49(8):1296–1307

80. Schramm J, Aliashkevich AF (2008) Temporal mediobasal tumors: a proposal for classification according to surgical anatomy. Acta Neurochir 150:857–864

81. Schwartzkroin PA, Walsh CA (2000) Cortical malformations and epilepsy. Ment Retard Dev Disabil Res Rev 6(4):268–280

82. Sinclair DB, Aronyk K, Snyder T, McKean J, Wheatley M, Bhargava R, Hoskinson M, Hao C, Colmers W (2003) Pediatric temporal lobectomy for epilepsy. Pediatr Neurosurg 38(4):195–205

83. Sinclair DB, Wheatley M, Aronyk K, Hao C, Snyder T, Colmers W, McKean JD (2001) Pathology and neuroimaging in pediatric temporal lobectomy for intractable epilepsy. Pediatr Neurosurg 35:239–246

84. Smith AP, Sani S, Kanner AM, Stoub T, Morrin M, Palac S, Bergen DC, Balabonov A, Smith M, Whisler WW, Byrne RW (2011) Medically intractable temporal lobe epilepsy in patients with normal MRI: surgical outcome in twenty-one consecutive patients. Seizure 20(6):475–479

85. Smith JR, VanderGriff A, Fountas K (2004) Temporal lobotomy in the surgical management of epilepsy: technical report. Neurosurgery 54(6):1531–1534

86. Smyth MD, Limbrick DD Jr, Ojemann JG, Zempel J, Robinson S, O'Brien DF, Saneto RP, Goyal M, Appleton RE, Mangano FT, Park TS (2007) Outcome following surgery for tempo-

ral lobe epilepsy with hippocampal involvement in preadolescent children: emphasis on mesial temporal sclerosis. J Neurosurg 106(3 Suppl):205–210

87. Sotero de Menezes MA, Connolly M, Bolanos A, Madsen J, Black PM, Riviello JJ Jr (2001) Temporal lobectomy in early childhood: the need for long-term follow-up. J Child Neurol 16(8):585–590

88. Spencer DD, Spencer SS, Mattson RH, Williamson PD, Novelly RA (1984) Access to the posterior medial temporal lobe structures in the surgical treatment of temporal lobe epilepsy. Neurosurgery 15(5):667–671

89. Spooner CG, Berkovic SF, Mitchell LA, Wrennall JA, Harvey AS (2006) New-onset temporal lobe epilepsy in children: lesion on MRI predicts poor seizure outcome. Neurology 67(12):2147–2153

90. Szabo CA, Wyllie E, Stanford LD, Geckler C, Kotagal P, Comair YG, Thornton AE (1998) Neuropsychological effect of temporal lobe resection in preadolescent children with epilepsy. Epilepsia 39:814–819

91. Sztriha L, Gururaj AK, Bener A, Nork M (2002) Temporal lobe epilepsy in children: etiology in a cohort with new-onset seizures. Epilepsia 43(1):75–80

92. Tanriverdi T, Olivier A (2007) Cognitive changes after unilateral cortico-amygdalohippocampectomy unilateral selective-amygdalohippocampectomy mesial temporal lobe epilepsy. Turk Neurosurg 17(2):91–99

93. Tezer FI, Akalan N, Oguz KK, Karabulut E, Dericioglu N, Ciger A, Saygi S (2008) Predictive factors for postoperative outcome in temporal lobe epilepsy according to two different classifications. Seizure 17(6):549–560

94. Tezer FI, Dericioglu N, Bozkurt G, Bilginer B, Akalan N, Saygi S (2011) Epilepsy surgery in patients with unilateral mesial temporal sclerosis and contralateral scalp ictal onset. Turk Neurosurg 21(4):549–554

95. Tonini C, Beghi E, Berg AT, Bogliun G, Giordano L, Newton RW, Tetto A, Vitelli E, Vitezic D, Wiebe S (2004) Predictors of epilepsy surgery outcome: a meta-analysis. Epilepsy Res 62:75–87

96. Usui N, Mihara T, Baba K, Matsuda K, Tottori T, Umeoka S, Nakamura F, Terada K, Usui K, Inoue Y (2008) Intracranial EEG findings in patients with lesional lateral temporal lobe epilepsy. Epilepsy Res 78(1):82–91

97. Wiebe S, Blume WT, Girvin JP, Eliasziw M (2001) A randomized, controlled trial of surgery for temporal-lobe epilepsy. N Engl J Med 345:311–318

98. Wieshmann UC, Larkin D, Varma T, Eldridge P (2008) Predictors of outcome after temporal lobectomy for refractory temporal lobe epilepsy. Acta Neurol Scand 118(5):306–312

99. Wyllie E, Chee M, Granström ML, DelGiudice E, Estes M, Comair Y, Pizzi M, Kotagal P, Bourgeois B, Lüders H (1993) Temporal lobe epilepsy in early childhood. Epilepsia 34:859–868

Treatment Modalities for Intractable Epilepsy in Hypothalamic Hamartoma

Joong-Uhn Choi and Dong-Seok Kim

Contents

Abstract Hypothalamic hamartoma (HH) is usually associated with refractory epilepsy, cognitive impairment, and behavioral disturbance. There is now increasing evidence that HH can be treated effectively with a variety of neurosurgical approaches. Treatment options for intractable gelastic seizure in HH patients include direct open surgery with craniotomy, endoscopic surgery, radiosurgery with gamma knife (GKS) and stereotactic radiofrequency thermocoagulation. Selection of treatment modalities depends on type and size of the HH and the surgeon's preference. Two surgical techniques, resection and disconnection, had been described with favorable outcomes. Pretreatment evaluation, patient selection, surgical techniques, complications, and possible selection of treatment are discussed in this chapter.

Keywords Hypothalamic hamartoma • Epilepsy • Gelastic seizure • Transcallosal resection • Endoscopic surgery • Radiosurgery • Stereotactic radiofrequency ablation

J.-U. Choi, M.D., Ph.D. (✉)
Department of Neurosurgery, CHA Bundang Medical Center, CHA University,
Sungnam, Gyeonggi-do, Korea
e-mail: juchoi@cha.ac.kr, juchoi@yuhs.ac

D.-S. Kim, M.D., Ph.D.
Department of Neurosurgery, Severance Hospital, Yonsei University Seoul, Korea
e-mail: dskim33@yuhs.ac

N. Akalan, C. Di Rocco (eds.), *Pediatric Epilepsy Surgery*,
Advances and Technical Standards in Neurosurgery,
DOI 10.1007/978-3-7091-1360-8_5, © Springer-Verlag Wien 2012

Introduction

Hypothalamic hamartomas (HHs) are rare congenital non-neoplastic lesions of the inferior hypothalamus and consist of an abnormal mixture of neuronal and glial tissue. They issue from the floor of the third ventricle, tuber cinereum, or mammillary bodies. Hypothalamic hamartoma can be classified as sessile or pedunculated, depending on the width of their attachment to hypothalamus. Various symptoms have been associated with the sessile type of HH, including refractory epilepsy, central precocious puberty, intellectual impairment, and behavioral problems [10].

Epilepsy appears in early childhood and quickly becomes refractory to medical treatment. Gelastic seizures represent the most common clinical expression of epilepsy and cause the patient to present sudden, brief, uncontrollable attacks of laughter. These gelastic attacks progress as the patient ages, and other types of seizure, cognitive deterioration, and behavioral problems appear, frequently developing late in first decade of life, together with drop attacks and other secondary generalized epilepsy symptoms [2].

It has been demonstrated that epileptic focus originates from the hamartoma and from neocortical foci strictly related to HHs.

Preoperative Evaluation and Patient Selection

Presurgical evaluation includes routine electroencephalographic (EEG) monitoring and video-EEG monitoring with scalp electrodes, interictal and ictal 99m-Tc hexamethylprophyleneamine oxime single photon emission computed tomography (SPECT), magnetic resonance imaging (MRI), neuropsychological evaluation, ophthalmological assessments with perimetry, and endocrinological investigations.

The dimensions of the HHs and the anatomy surrounding the tuber cinereum can be seen clearly by high-resolution coronal and sagittal T1-weighted MRI. Endocrine assessment includes measurement of basal gonadotrophin and growth hormone levels, thyroid function, prolactin level, and cortisol reserve with glucagon stimulation. Deep electrode insertion into the HH with EEG monitoring may be necessary in some cases.

Intractable seizure of the predominant gelastic type is an indication for surgical treatment. Gelastic seizures refractory to medication, neurobehavioral deterioration and direct or indirect evidence of hypothalamic seizure origin, and the absence of a cortical lesion on MRI are recommended for surgical treatment. The potential risks to memory, endocrine function, behavior, and vision have to be explained to the parents.

Treatments

Since Paillas et al. reported successful seizure outcome after resection of HHs in some patients in 1969, surgical intervention for these lesions has been attempted with variable seizure outcome [2]. Four surgical treatments have been introduced to treat HH: direct open surgery with craniotomy, endoscopic surgery, radiosurgery with gamma knife (GKS), and stereotactic radiofrequency thermocoagulation. Two techniques for HH surgery are used: resection or disconnection of hamartoma. The concept of disconnection had been introduced by Delalande and Fohlin [4] and it showed dramatic improvement in the patient. The technique disconnects the connecting tract between the hamartoma and the surrounding normal tissue.

Open Surgery with Craniotomy

Multiple surgical approaches to the resection of HH have been described. Transbasal approaches with variations, such as the standard pterional approach, extended pterional approach with orbitotomy, and subfrontal approach, were reported but unfortunately many of these techniques were associated with high complication rates, including infarction of the internal capsule and thalamus, cranial nerve palsy (third nerve, olfactory nerve, and optic nerve), endocrinopathy, and memory loss. There also were difficulties in completely excising the lesion which extended into third ventricle.

Delalande and Fohlen [4] introduced disconnecting surgical treatment for extraventricular HH in 2003. Dramatic improvement in 53 % of those who underwent the procedure using pterional approach was reported. Two of 14 disconnection surgeries showed ischemic complications.

Rosenfeld et al. reported their experience with the transcallosal interforniceal approach in 2000 [16]. Complete or nearly complete resection of HHs can be safely achieved via this approach with the possibility of seizure freedom and neurobehavioral improvement.

Transcallosal Interforniceal Approach

Surgical Technique

The patient is placed under general anesthesia in the supine position, with the neck well flexed so that the head is horizontal and fixed in the three-pin headrest. A small frontoparietal craniotomy with the best trajectory to the HH is chosen using a neuronavigation system. Using the microscope, the right hemisphere is gently retracted from the falx and an opening (2–3 cm) is made in the anterior portion of the body of the corpus callosum, with the protection of the pericallosal vessels. Using neuronavigation guidance to remain in the midline, an interforniceal approach is used to enter the roof of the third ventricle, minimizing retraction of the fornices. The cavum septum pellucidum is transverse if it is present, The lateral wall of the third ventricle is used as the limit of resection. The long microsurgery instruments, including bipolar forceps, sucker, and microscissors, have to be prepared. It also is helpful to use an ultrasonic aspirator with a long microtip and long microaspirators. The limit of lateral resection is the normal third ventricular wall and resection is extended inferiorly to the translucent third ventricle floor. The surgeon must take care to minimize trauma to the mammillary bodies.

The transcallosal approach is technically more difficult and hazardous to perform in children less than 18 months of age due to the narrow third ventricle. Also, patients with large HHs that extend beneath the third ventricle floor will not be a good candidate for this approach [16].

Results and Complications

Rosenfeld et al. reported complete or near total resection (>95 %) of HH in about 62 % of the patients and 75–95 % resection was possible in about 24 % of the patients [16].

Harvey et al. reported that transcallosal resection of HH was effective treatment for intractable epilepsy, with 54–76 % of the patients being seizure-free or having a >90 % reduction in seizures. There also were improvements in behavior and cognition in 65–88 %. With univariate analysis, the likelihood of a seizure-free outcome correlated with younger age, shorter lifetime duration of epilepsy, smaller volume of HH, and complete HH resection [7].

Postoperative complications were stroke, short-term memory disturbance, weight gain, diabetes insipidus, and other endocrine disturbances. Stroke is probably the result of injury of perforating vessels surrounding HH and short-term memory disturbance is due to surgical trauma of the septal, forniceal, or mammillary body. Endocrinological morbidity is likely due to injury of neurovascular structure or pituitary stalk.

Injuries to the optic tract and cranial nerve were rare with the transcallosal approach, but these injuries have been reported with the traditional pterional and subfrontal approaches [11].

Endoscopic Surgery

Classification of HH and Indication

Choi et al. [3] modified classification of sessile HH, which was proposed by Delalande and Fohlen [4] (Fig. 1). Small HHs (<20 mm) were classified as midline (Type I), lateral (Type II), or intraventricular (Type III) according to the location of the HH relative to the hypothalamus and third ventricle. A large hamartoma (>20 mm) was defined as giant HH (Type IV).

Delalande and Fohlen first reported on the use of endoscopic disconnection only for intraventricular type of hamartoma (Type III) in 2003 [4]. They also did endoscopic procedures in addition to conventional open surgery to treat other types of hamartoma. However, Choi et al. [3] had tried endoscopic disconnection for Type I, Type II, and Type III as the primary option of treatment and also used endoscopic surgery as an additional procedure for Type IV HH.

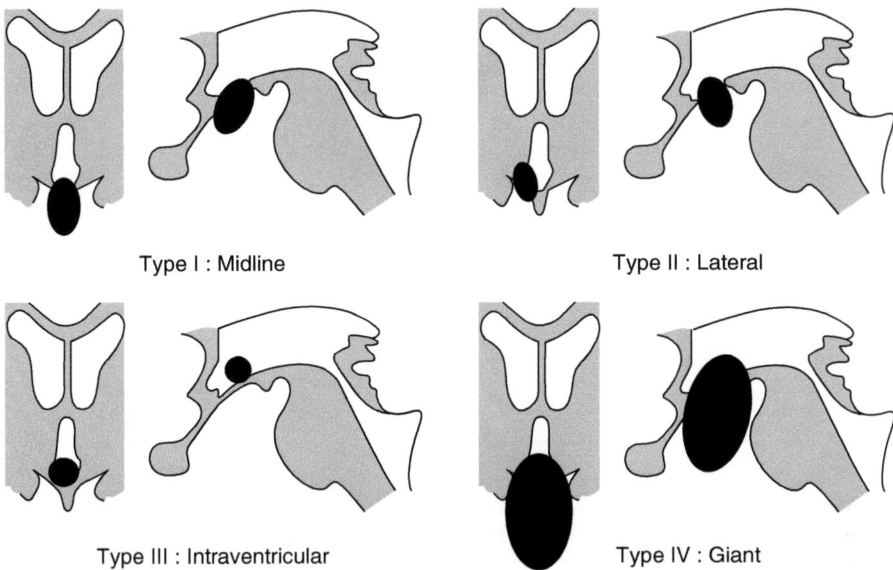

Fig. 1 Classification of sessile hypothalamic hamartoma (HH) (Modified by Choi et al. [3] from that proposed by Delalande and Fohlen [4]). The HHs were divided into four categories based on MR imaging findings demonstrating the relationship between the hamartoma and hypothalamus or the third ventricle. A large hamartoma (>20 mm) was defined as a giant HH (Type IV). Small HHs (<20 mm) were classified as midline (Type I), lateral (Type II), and intraventricular (Type III) according to their relative location to the third ventricle

Surgical Technique

The instrumentation for endoscopic disconnection consists of a 30° Hopkins pediatric telescope (Karl Storz GmbH &Co., Tuttingen, Germany) with an outside diameter 2.7 mm, a sheath for the telescope with outside diameter of 3.8 mm, a stylet, a monopolar electric coagulator or Nd-YAG laser system, forceps, a fiberoptic light guide, a Xe light source, and an endovision system. An endoscopic procedure is performed after induction of general anesthesia. In the standard procedure, a burr hole is made 1 cm in front of the coronal suture and 2–3 cm lateral to the midline. For a lateral type of HH (Type II), a contralateral approach gives better visualization of the hamartoma and makes the disconnection procedure easier. The lateral ventricle is tapped using a ventricular catheter through the burr hole. Neuronavigation is helpful in making the ventricular tap because the size of the ventricles is normal in most patients. After successful tapping, a peel-away catheter is then replaced via the tract. The telescope with the sheath is then advanced into the lateral ventricle through the peel-away catheter. When the telescope is advanced into the third ventricle via the foramen of Monro, the surgeon can see the HH protruding from the floor and lateral wall of the third ventricle. With the lateral type (Type II) or the intraventricular type (Type III) of HH, it will be easier to

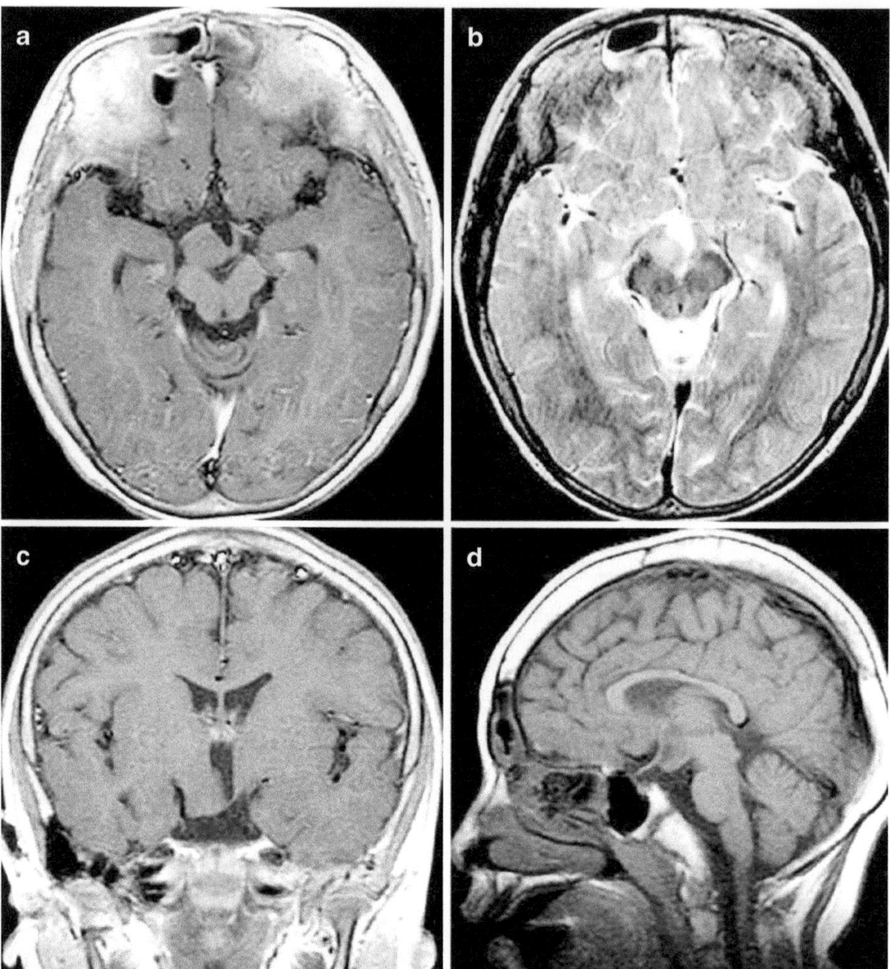

Fig. 2 (**a**) T1-weighted axial image showing a round, nonenhanced, isointense mass attached to the hypothalamus on the right side. It seems to be attached to the mammillary body and the tuber cinereum posteriorly. (**b**) T2-weighted image showing that the mass has a slightly bright signal intensity. (**c**) T1-weighted coronal image showing the mass extending from the hypothalamus and ambiguous differentiation from the hypothalamus. (**d**) T1-weighted sagittal image showing the location of the mass adjacent to the tuber cinereum and between the optic chiasm and mammillary body

define the HH margin by comparing the normal side of the third ventricle wall. However, for the midline type (Type I) of HH, the surgeon sometimes can have difficulty determining the HH margin. The main site of endoscopic disconnection will be along the midline posteroinferior floor and lateral wall of the third ventricle. The surgeon has to take care not to injure the mammillary body and normal hypothalamic tissue along the third ventricle wall. The depth of disconnection is determined by examining the preoperative T1- and T2-weighted coronal MR images (Fig. 2). For disconnection, the monopolar electric coagulator or fiber-optic electrode of the Nd-YAG laser system is advanced through the working channel of the sheath and severs or coagulates the HH along the planned margin. The planned margin (mapping) is made by surface coagulation initially and the disconnection proceeds under direct vision (Fig. 3).

In deepening the disconnection, some part of the HH can be removed by forceps in order to see the surgical field of coagulation. The roles of neuronavigation and direct visualization are important in checking the depth of disconnection (Fig. 4). Depending on the anatomy of the individual hamartoma, the interface is dissected until the pial surface or the ependymal surface of the floor of third ventricle is identified. Postoperatively, disconnection of the HH from the hypothalamus can be confirmed by air density along the disconnection site on brain CT or by signal changes on T1- and T2-weighted coronal MR images (Fig. 5).

Results and Complications

Shim et al. [18] (the authors' group) reported their experience with endoscopic disconnection in 11 patients in 2008. Six of 11 patients were seizure-free (Engel's class 1) immediately after surgery. Improvement in behavior was also noted in these patients after 2 months. Outcome in three patients was class 2. In two other complicated cases which were treated with gamma knife surgery previously, seizure control was not satisfactory (class 3 or 4), but most cases showed complete resolution or a reduction of gelastic seizures.

Procaccini et al. (the Delalande group) reported the results of 13 patients treated with frameless stereotactic endoscopic surgery in 2006 [13]. Seizure-free recovery (Engel class 1) was achieved in 54 % of the patients, and 46 % of the patients showed improvement (Engel class 3). For the intraventricular type of HH, 90 % of patients became seizure-free postoperatively.

Rekate et al. [15] reported their experience with endoscopic removal in 44 patients based on early results.

Ideal candidates for this surgery are those with a lesion smaller than 1.5 cm in diameter. Patients with larger lesions also may be candidates as long as 6 mm of clearance is present to the top of the third ventricle. In Rekate's series, early complications occurred in 11 (25 %) of 44 patients but resolved within 3 months in all but three patients (6.8 %), including one patient with postoperative hemiparesis and two patients with short-term memory loss. Early complications included transient short-term memory loss, weight gain, thalamic infarction with memory loss, and hemiparesis [9, 15].

Choi et al. [3] observed postoperative disconnection-like syndrome in three patients, which included mental dullness, verbal anomia, unilateral tactile anomia, and lack of somesthetic transfer. This disconnection-like syndrome disappeared spontaneously within 10 days.

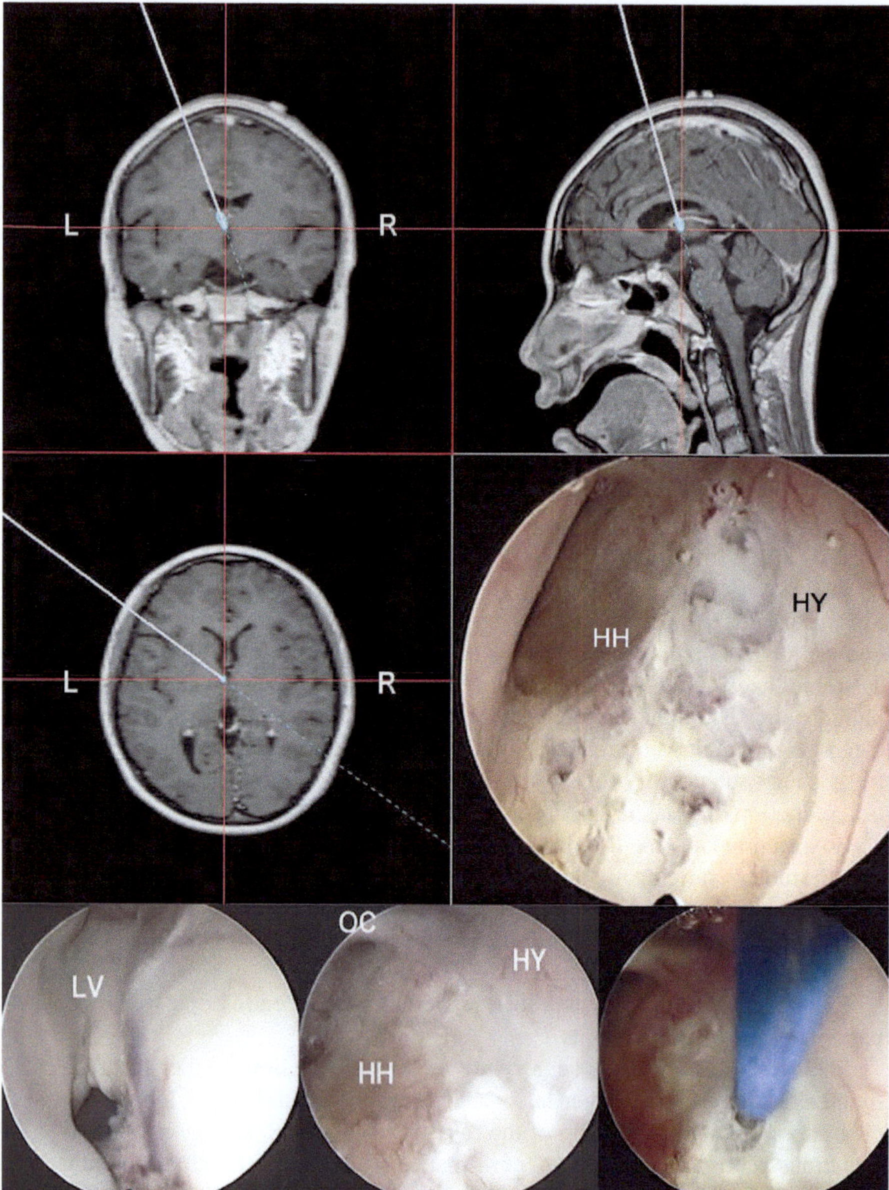

Fig. 3 Views captured during neuronavigation for endoscopic disconnection. Because the main connection between the hypothalamic hamartoma (*HH*) and the hypothalamus was on the right side, the initial approach was started through a left frontal burr hole. As the image shows, the trajectory toward the interface between the HH and the hypothalamus could be easily determined. The lower-right photograph captured by the endoscope showed the initial site of the disconnection. The three photographs at the bottom were captured during endoscopic disconnection. Under guidance of neuronavigation, the left lateral ventricle was entered and the foramen of Monro was seen. The interface between the HH and the hypothalamus could be delineated with direct visualization and the assistance of neuronavigation. With a unipolar coagulator, disconnection was successfully performed. *R* right, *L* left, *OC* optic chiasm, *HY* hypothalamus, *LV* left lateral ventricle

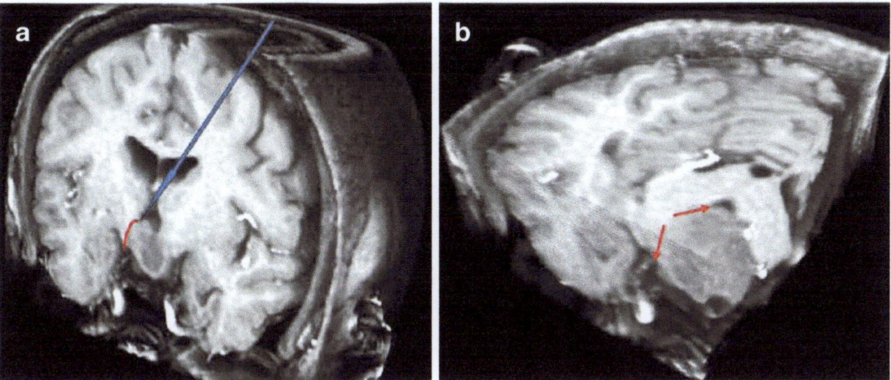

Fig. 4 Three-dimensional illustrations showing the endoscopic disconnection procedure. (**a**) The neuronavigation system could determine the initial approach trajectory (*blue line*) and initial disconnection site. (**b**) Further disconnection proceeded toward the basal cistern and interpeduncular cistern (*red arrows*)

Radiosurgery

Destruction of the HH lesion using focused ionizing radiation (gamma knife) is an attractive approach that does not require invasive surgery. Although a delayed (4–6 months) response to gamma knife treatment is expected, early results suggest variable outcomes. Regis et al. [14] reported excellent early seizure response. However, results in terms of long-term seizure freedom are not clear.

The treatment goal of radiosurgery for HH is to deliver doses high enough to affect epileptogenesis without exceeding the tolerance of nearby critical structures. Modern radiosurgical devices such as Gamma Knife (Elekta AG), Cyber Knife (Accuray Inc.), and Novalis (BrainLab AG) can deliver conformal high-dose radiation with steep gradients providing a chance to achieve seizure freedom without hypothalamic or cranial nerve damage. Achievement of an excellent outcome following radiosurgery is related to the dose delivered. Regis et al. [14] observed that four patients who received a peripheral dose of 18 Gy with the Gamma Knife became seizure free. Careful treatment planning and very tight dose distribution are essential to delivering similar doses without injuring the optic chiasm, optic tracts, pituitary stalk, fornices, mammillary bodies, and hypothalamic nuclei.

The mean size of HH in a large series of radiosurgery was 19 mm in diameter, but radiosurgery can be accomplished in lesions smaller than 30 mm by using steep dose gradients around the target [14].

No serious complication have been reported with radiosurgery but temporary worsening of seizures can be seen as early as 2 months after the procedure.

Successful radiosurgical treatment of epileptogenic HHs was first reported in 1998 by Arita and colleagues [1]. Regis et al. [14] found a clear correlation between dose and efficacy; the marginal dose was >17 Gy in all patients in whom seizure freedom was achieved and all patients who received <13 Gy showed incomplete

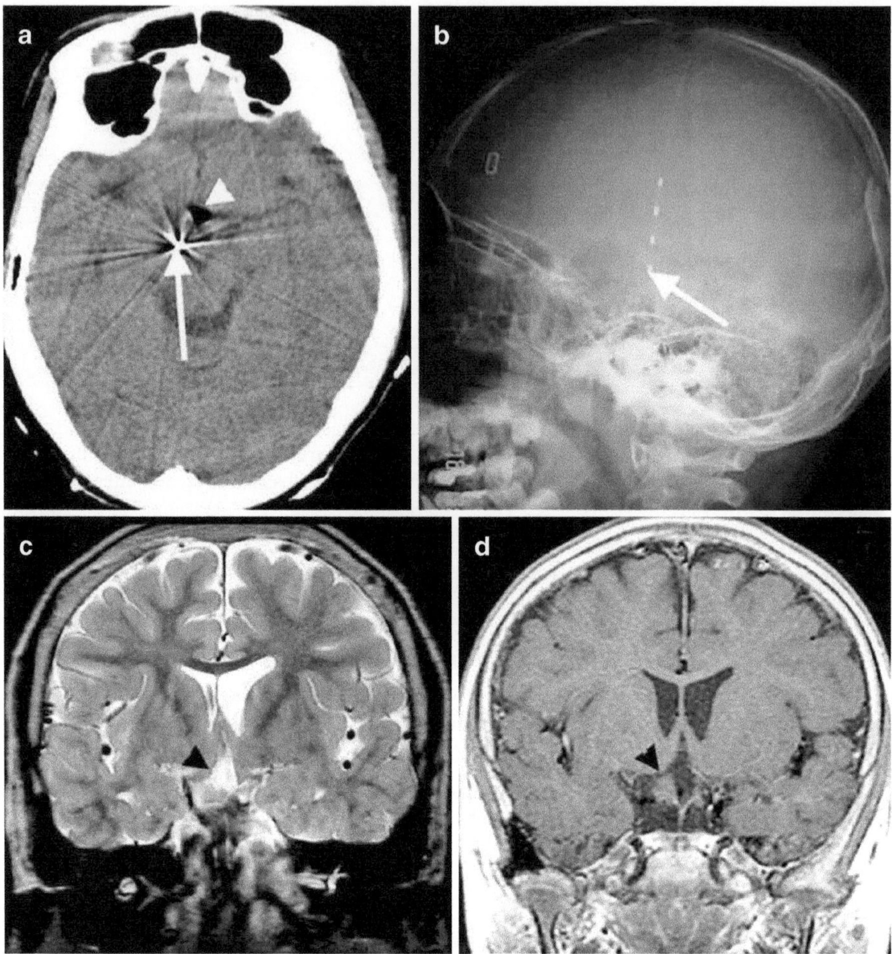

Fig. 5 Postoperative neuroimaging study. (**a**) Postoperative computed tomography scan showing air density in the prepontine cistern (*white arrowhead*), which means complete fenestration between the third ventricle and the prepontine cistern by neuroendoscopy, and artifacts (*arrow*) resulting from the depth electrode in the hypothalamic hamartoma. (**b**) The lateral view of the cranial X-ray revealing the depth electrode in the hypothalamic hamartoma. (**c, d**) T2- and T1-weighted coronal MRI scans demonstrating the disconnection between the mass (*arrowheads*) and the hypothalamus

seizure control. Updated outcome of a large series (over 60 patients) by Regis et al. showed that 40 % were seizure free (Engel class 1) and 20 % of the patients had fewer seizures. However, in the other series in which doses ranging from 12 to 14 Gy were used, outcome of seizure control was variable [17, 18].

Radiosurgery can be a safe, effective, and noninvasive first-line treatment for small epileptogenic HHs [14].

Stereotactic Radiofrequency Ablation

In 1999 Fukuda et al. [6] reported on a single patient with HH treated by stereotactic radiofrequency thermocoagulation in the course of exploration with a depth electrode implanted within the lesion. Gelastic seizures ceased postoperatively and tonic seizures disappeared 4 months later. Finally, this patient became seizure free within 14 months.

Surgical Technique

To confirm epileptic discharges from the hamartoma, depth electrode recording could be obtained by means of a chronically implanted electrode. With the patient under local and intravenous propofol anesthesia, the Leksell stereotactic frame (Elekta, Sweden) is attached to the patient's head. A quadripolar deep brain electrode (3387; Medtronic) is inserted into the hamartoma through frontal burr holes. The depth electrode consists of four contacts (with contact 0 the most ventral and contact 3 the most dorsal), which are 1.3 mm in diameter, 1.5 mm long, and 1.5 mm apart. The target within hamartoma is determined by MRI-based software (Leksell SurgiPlan, Elekta) or the neuronavigational system. Epileptic discharges are detected by implanted depth electrodes in the hamartoma. Video-EEG recording can be used during monitoring for some period.

Thermocoagulation can be performed after or without depth electrode recording. With the patient under local and intravenous propofol anesthesia, the Leksell stereotactic frame is applied to patient's head and three-dimensional reconstruction of MR images confirm the spatial relationship between the HH and the surrounding neural structures such as the optic tracts, internal capsules, and hypothalamus. Electrode entry points, trajectories, and targets are determined to avoid damaging these critical structures and ventricles. One or several targets through two to five trajectories are planned to ablate the HH according to its size. For depth electrode recording, the depth electrodes are replaced with coagulation needles 2 mm in diameter and with a 4-mm uninsulated tip at the same depth as the electrodes. After discontinuation of intravenous propofol anesthesia, test heating (60 °C, 30 s) is performed to determine whether major complications are likely to occur. If patients do not experience any complications during the test, then lesions can be made (74 °C, 60 s). Thermocoagulation could be performed under general anesthesia in patients with severe mental retardation.

Results and Complications

Homma et al. [8] reported the results of five cases treated with stereotactic radiofrequency thermocoagulation in 2007. Four of five patients (80 %) were free of gelastic seizures by the time of final examination, although one patient required two surgeries. Three of four patients were free not only from gelastic seizures but also from other types of seizures, whereas the fourth patient continued to experience other types of seizures at decreased frequency.

Complications included low-grade fever (4 patients) and hyperphagia (2 patients) and occurred transiently as local hypothalamic symptoms. These transient symptoms resolved within 1 week after surgery after perifocal edema disappeared; no permanent complications were noted. This procedure seems to be effective for a small hamartoma but a long-term study of a large series will be necessary to confirm the efficacy and safety of this treatment [5, 8, 12].

Selection of Treatment

Selection of the neurosurgical procedure to perform depends on the surgeon's preference and experience, but reasonable approaches can be selected according to the location, shape, and size of the HH. Possible treatment selections according to

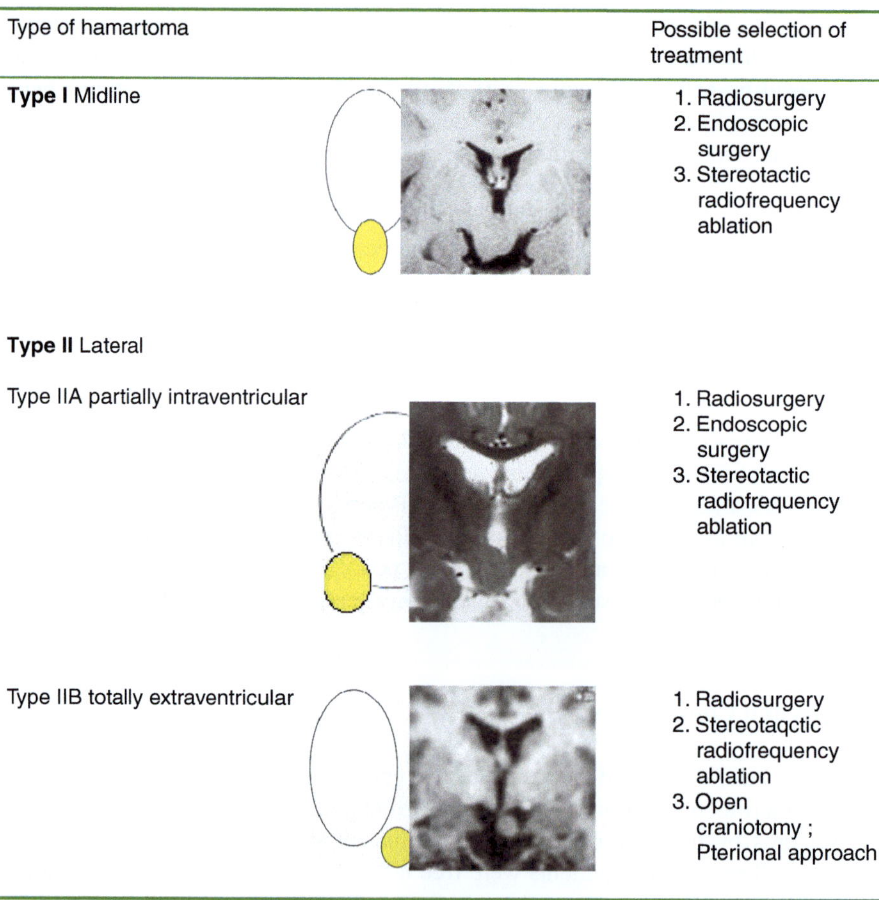

Fig. 6 Possible treatments for subdivided types of hypothalamic hamartoma (modification from Choi's [3] and Delalande and Fohlen's [4] classification)

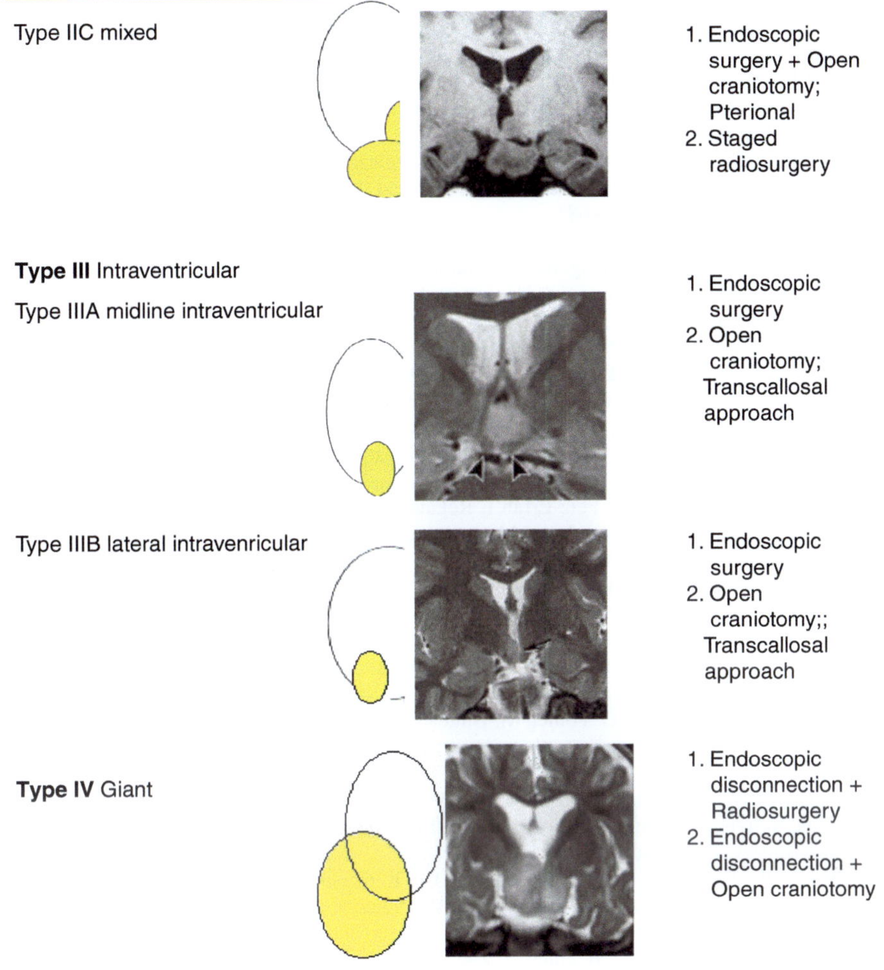

Fig. 6 (continued)

subdivided types of hypothalamic hamartoma are given in Fig 6, although treatment options can be different depending on the viewpoint of the surgeon.

Acknowledgments The authors thank Professor Tae-Gon Kim and Miss Sang-Hee Ahn for their help in preparing the manuscript.

References

1. Arita K, Kurisu K, Iida K, Hanaya R, Akimitsu T, Hibino S et al (1998) Subsidence of seizure induced by stereotactic radiation in a patient with hypothalamic hamartoma. Case report. J Neurosurg 89:645–648

2. Berkovic SF, Arzimanoglou A, Kuzniecky R, Harvey AS, Palmini A, Andermann F (2003) Hypothalamic hamartoma and seizure: a treatable epileptic encephalopathy. Epilepsia 4:969–973
3. Choi JU, Yang KH, Kim TG, Chang JH, Chang JW, Lee BI, Kim DS (2004) Endoscopic disconnection for hypothalamic hamartoma with intractable seizure. Report of four cases. J Neurosurg 100:506–511
4. Delalande O, Fohlen M (2003) Disconnecting surgical treatment of hypothalamic hamartoma in children and adults with refractory epilepsy and proposal of a new classification. Neurol Med Chir (Tokyo) 43(2):61–68
5. Fujimoto Y, Kato A, Saitoh Y, Ninomiya H, Imai K, Hashimoto N et al (2005) Open radiofrequency ablation for the management of intractable epilepsy associated with sessile hypothalamic hamartoma. Minim Invasive Neurosurg 48(3):132–135
6. Fukuda M, Kameyama S, Wachi M, Tanka R (1999) Stereotxy for hypothalamic hamartoma with intractable gelastic seizures: Technical case report. Neurosurgery 44:1347–1350
7. Harvey AS, Freeman JL, Berkovic SF, Rosenfeld JV (2003) Transcallosal resection of hypothalamic hamartomas in patients with intractable epilepsy. Epileptic Disord 5(4):257–265
8. Homma J, Kameyama S, Masuda H, Ueno T, Fujimoto A, Oishi M, Fukuda M (2007) Stereotactic radiofrequency thermocoagulation for hypothalamic hamartoma with intractable gelastic seizures. Epilepsy Res 76:15–21
9. Lekovic GP, Gonzalez LF, Feiz-Erfan I, Rekate H (2006) Endoscopic resection of hypothalamic hamartoma using a novel variable aspiration tissue resector. Neurosurgery 58:166–169
10. Likavec AM, Dickerman RD, Heiss JD, Liow K (2000) Retrospective analysis of surgical treatment outcomes for gelastic seizures: a review of the literature. Seizure 9(3):204–207
11. Ng YT, Rekate HL, Prenger EC, Chung SS, Feiz-Erfan I, Wang NC et al (2006) Transcallosal resection of hypothalamic hamartoma for intractable epilepsy. Epilepsia 47(7):1192–1202
12. Parrent AG (1999) Stereotactic radiofrequency ablation for the treatment of gelastic seizures associated with hypothalamic hamartoma. Case report. J Neurosurg 91(5):881–884
13. Procaccini E, Dorfmuller G, Fohlen M, Bulteau C, Delalande O (2006) Surgical management of hypothalamic hamartomas with epilepsy: the stereoendoscopic approach. Neurosurgery 59:336–345
14. Régis J, Scavarda D, Tamura M, Nagayi M, Villeneuve N, Bartolomei F et al (2006) Epilepsy related to hypothalamic hamartomas: surgical management with special reference to gamma knife surgery. J Neurosurg 104(6):913–924
15. Rekate HL, Feiz-Erfan I, Ng YT, Gonzalez LF, Kerrigan JF (2006) Endoscopic surgery for hypothalamic hamartomas causing medically refractory gelastic epilepsy. Childs Nerv Syst 22(8):874–880
16. Rosenfeld JV, Harvey AS, Wrennall J, Zacharin M, Berkovic SF (2001) Transcallosal resection of hypothalamic hamartomas, with control of seizures, in children with gelastic epilepsy. Neurosurgery 48(1):108–118
17. Schulze-Bonhage A, Homberg V, Trippel M, Keimer R, Elger CE, Warnke PC et al (2004) Interstitial radiosurgery in the treatment of gelastic epilepsy due to hypothalamic hamartomas. Neurology 62(4):644–647
18. Shim KW, Chang JH, Park YG, Kim HD, Choi JU, Kim DS (2008) Treatment modality for intractable epilepsy in hypothalamic hamartomatous lesions. Neurosurgery 62:847–856

Epilepsy in Tuberous Sclerosis Complex

Federica Novegno, Luca Massimi, and Concezio Di Rocco

Contents

Abstract Tuberous Sclerosis Complex (TSC) is an autosomal dominant multisystem disorder, characterized by the presence of hamartomatous lesions involving different organ systems, including the brain. Epilepsy is the most common presenting symptom, representing a major source of morbidity and mortality. Despite multiple antiepileptic drug combinations, in about two thirds of cases the patients present high-frequency drug-resistant epilepsy, and nonpharmacologic options may be considered. The aim of this work was to point out the current knowledge on epileptogenesis in TSC, the available medical therapies and diagnostic tools, and possible surgical strategies, with the intent to better understand the actual difficulties in controlling seizures and the results reported in the literature. There is also a section

F. Novegno, M.D. (✉) • L. Massimi, M.D. • C. Di Rocco, M.D.
Department of Pediatric Neurosurgery, Catholic University Medical School,
Largo A. Gemelli 1, 00168 Rome, Italy
e-mail: federicanovegno@hotmail.it

N. Akalan, C. Di Rocco (eds.), *Pediatric Epilepsy Surgery*,
Advances and Technical Standards in Neurosurgery,
DOI 10.1007/978-3-7091-1360-8_6, © Springer-Verlag Wien 2012

dedicated to the common association with cognitive impairment and the role of epilepsy control on its outcome.

Keywords Tuberous sclerosis complex • Epilepsy surgery • Epileptogenesis

General Features

Tuberous Sclerosis Complex (TSC) is a genetic multisystem disorder, dominantly inherited, with high penetrance but variably expressed. It is characterized by the presence of hamartomas (tumor-like masses) involving different organ systems. It is the third most common neurocutaneous syndrome, following Pascual-Castroviejo type II syndrome (P-CIIS) or PHACE association and neurofibromatosis I [92, 93, 101].

The term tuberous sclerosis was introduced a century ago to describe the potato-like consistency of cortical gyri with hypertrophic sclerosis found at autopsy over the brain of patients who had suffered mental delay and seizures [15].

TSC incidence is estimated to be as high as 1 in 5,800 live births [23, 89], with a prevalence at 1 in 10,000 [86], although its true incidence is supposed to be underestimated because of a number of undiagnosed cases, mainly of mildly affected or asymptomatic patients.

Pathophysiology

TSC is an autosomal dominant disorder, although two thirds of patients present a sporadic mutation. TSC is caused by the inactivating mutations in either of two genes, *TSC1* (located on chromosome 9q34, encoding for hamartin) and *TSC2* (located on chromosome 16p13.3, encoding for tuberin). About 350 different mutations in both TSC genes have been described [85]. The mutation spectra of these genes are very heterogeneous and no preferred sites of mutation have been reported (hotspots): indeed, they are distributed over the entire regions of both genes, comprising nonsense, missense, insertion, and deletion mutations. In about 10–15 % of cases, no mutations have been identified [32].

Hamartin and tuberin are proteins coexpressed in cells of different organs such as kidney, lung, brain, and pancreas. *TSC1* and *TSC2* mRNA and protein have been observed in cerebral cortex, hippocampus, cerebellum, brainstem, choroid plexum epithelium, and spinal cord of the immature and mature brain [86].

They form a GAP complex (a GTPase-activating protein) that inhibits the mammalian target of rapamycin (mTOR) signaling cascade and the associated kinase signaling cascades and translational factors, which results in increased cell growth and proliferation [21, 32, 50, 81, 85]. Mutations to either *TSC1* or *TSC2* compromise the function of the complex, so that mutations to either gene cause the same disease [85].

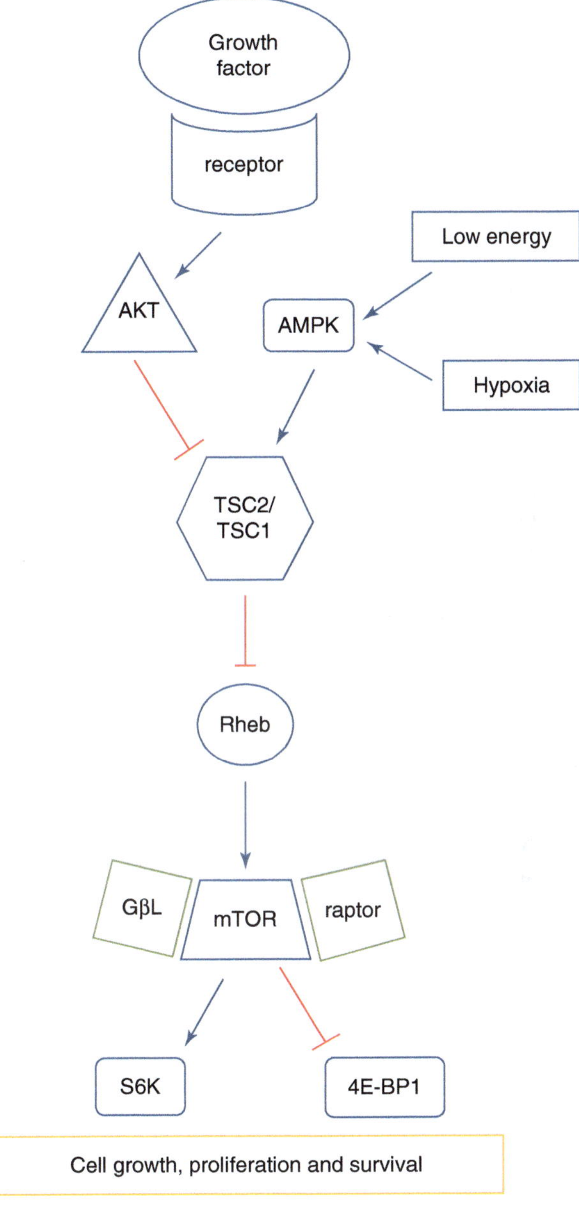

Fig. 1 Schematic description of mTOR signaling cascade. *AKT* protein kinase B, *AMPK* 5′ adenosine monophosphate-activated protein kinase, *Rheb* Ras-related superfamily of small G-proteins, *S6k1* ribosomal protein S6 kinase beta-1, *4E-BP1* eukaryotic translation initiation factor 4E-binding protein 1

Briefly (Fig. 1), after growth-factor stimulation, the TSC1/TSC2 protein complex is phosphorylated by AKT (protein kinase B), decreasing its GTPase-activating protein activity, whereas upon hypoxic or low-energy stimuli, the TSC1/TSC2 protein complex is phosphorylated by the AMPK 5′ adenosine monophosphate-activated protein kinase, increasing its GTPase-activating protein activity [32, 50].

Table 1 Revised diagnostic criteria for TSC (1998)

Major features	Minor features
Facial angiofibromas or forehead plaque	Multiple, randomly distributed pits in dental enamel
Nontraumatic ungual or periungual fibroma	Hamartomatous rectal polyps
Hypomelanotic macule (three or more)	Bone cysts: X-ray confirmation is sufficient
Shagreen patch (connective tissue nevus)	Cerebral white matter radial migration lines
Multiple retinal nodular hamartomas	Gingival fibromas
Cortical tubers	Nonrenal hamartomas
Subependymal nodules	Retinal achromic patch
Subependymal giant cell astrocytoma	"Confetti" skin lesions
Cardiac rhabdomyoma, single or multiple	Multiple renal cysts
Lymphangioleiomyomatosis	
Renal angiomyolipoma	

The TSC1/TSC2 protein complex inactivated by AKT inhibits the Rheb (Ras-related superfamily of small G proteins), which is the GTPase that activates the mTOR; the inactivation of the TSC1/TSC2 protein complex results in activation of mTOR. The mTOR is a serine-threonine kinase, bound to raptor and GβL, which regulates translation of p70S6 kinase and 4E-BP1, respectively, up- and downregulating their activities. The p70S6 kinase is the enzyme that phosphorylates the ribosomal protein S6 (S6k1) that induces ribosome biogenesis, and 4E-BP1 is an eukaryote initiation factor that acts as translational repressor; consequently, mTOR positively regulates protein synthesis, cell growth, and survival [50, 89].

Clinical Phenotype

The diagnosis of TSC is still based upon clinical grounds, but it may be challenging because no single symptom is present in all patients and none are absolutely pathognomonic. The specific diagnostic clinical criteria have been revised during the last two decades according to the recent advances in both clinical information and molecular genetics and have been simplified into two main categories based on the diagnostic importance and degree of specificity for TS of each clinical and radiological feature [29, 97, 102].

Once two major features or one major plus two minor features are demonstrated, the diagnosis of TSC may be established (Table 1). Early identification of TSC is vital because some serious clinical consequences may be prevented with a prompt diagnostic workup. Actually, despite the large number of clinical characteristics defined, diagnosis in early childhood, especially below 2 years of age, might be difficult because some stigmata become apparent only in late childhood or adulthood [60, 102, 104]. Recently, the availability of new molecular genetic testing has enabled a precocious diagnosis by detecting the mutation in either the *TSC1* or the *TSC2* gene in 75–80 % of cases.

Several genotype–phenotype studies have reported that as a group, TSC patients with a *TSC2* mutation have a more severe phenotype than those with a *TSC1* mutation [56].

Central Nervous System

Neurologic manifestations of TSC were first described by D.M. Bourneville in 1880, and in 1908 they were associated to clinical signs by H. Vogt, who first reported the "classic triad" of symptoms in TSC: seizures, mental delay, and adenoma sebaceum (angiofibromas). The characteristic brain lesions are represented by cortical tubers, subependymal nodules, subependymal giant cell astrocytomas (SEGAs), and radial myelinated tracts extending from subependymal areas to the cortex surface.

Epileptic Syndrome

Epilepsy is the most common presenting symptom in TSC and it represents a significant source of morbidity and mortality [13, 22, 29, 94, 109]. Data from literature report a prevalence of epilepsy in TSC up to 80–90 % [21, 23]. In the majority of cases, seizures occur in early childhood, especially during the first year of life, or even during the first months of life (two thirds of patients). The seizures are at first focal seizures, mainly partial motor seizures, which can coexist or develop, more frequently, into a cluster of spasms in infancy, or they may be followed by a secondary bilateral synchrony in late childhood [32, 81]. Rare cases of gelastic seizures have been reported [24]. Generally, the seizures originate in restricted areas, which may be localized, but generalization occurs frequently with bilateral diffusion and consequent generalized clinical manifestations [81]. An electroencephalography (EEG) may detect the presence of focal or multifocal epileptiform activities between the neonatal period and the occurrence of infantile spasms. However, subtle unilateral tonic or clonic phenomena, mainly involving the face or limbs, might be underrecognized by the relatives until they evolve into a typical cluster of spasms, especially upon awakening, by the third or fourth month of life. Lateralizing features, namely, tonic eye deviation, head turning, unilateral grimacing, and asymmetrical involvement of limbs can be observed [81].

There is a high incidence of infantile spasms and hypsarrhythmia in TSC, reported to be the presenting symptom in up to 69 % of patients, whereas TSC has been detected in 7–25 % of patients affected by West syndrome [28, 67]. However, the clinical and EEG findings in TSC patients with infantile spasms differ significantly from those with classical West syndrome. The infantile spasms observed in TSC patients appear earlier in comparison with other etiologies. Almost all the cases of infantile spasms in TSC occur between the end of the second and the 11th month of life, prevalently between the fourth and fifth month of life, rarely presenting before the third month. Infantile spasms associated with TSC often occur with a characteristic pattern, observed mainly in the early-onset cases: there is the presence of apparently bilateral and symmetrical flexor-tonic contractions of the limbs lasting for a few seconds and preceded by eye deviation [28]. Isolated attacks develop within weeks into the typical clusters, particularly while the infant is awakening. The atonic or tonic components presented in infantile spasms are often asymmetrical. The spasms may be unilateral with an adversative component.

In patients with TSC, the occurrence of a single seizure is likely to develop in epilepsy syndrome in nearly 100 %, and almost all the patients with infantile spasms develop another seizure phenotype, with multiple seizure types in half of them [21]. Despite the strong propensity for patients with TSC to develop epilepsy in childhood, more than 12% of adult patients affected by TSC without a previous history of seizures developed epilepsy, suggesting that patients affected by TSC remain at significant risk of epilepsy throughout their life [21].

Data from the literature reveal that patients with *TSC2* mutations have a higher frequency of epilepsy, and particularly have a greater risk of developing infantile spasms than those affected by *TSC1* mutations [21]. Familial cases are older at seizure onset than sporadic cases [56]. TSC patients with no identified mutation have a prevalent occurrence of infantile spasms but a significantly lower incidence of epilepsy when compared with patients with *TSC1* and *TSC2* mutations [16]. The more severe epileptic phenotype seems to be related to mutations that inactivate the GAP domain of tuberin (the *TSC2* product), which has been identified in cases with a greater cortical tuber load [57].

Electroencephalographic Findings

The characteristic EEG findings of TSC patients have been described accurately [23, 44, 115]. The majority of patients present epileptiform abnormalities (almost 80 %), whereas the remaining patients have slow-wave abnormalities or a normal EEG. Among the epileptiform abnormalities, focal spikes or sharp waves are detected in 35 % of cases, generalized epileptiform activities in 10 %, and hypsarrhythmia, with a disorganized background rhythm associated with multifocal slowing, multifocal epileptiform abnormalities, and paroxysmal attenuation of the background, can be observed in 22 % of cases. Ninety percent of patients with TSC show at least one region of consistent interictal epileptiform activity. Patients with one or two regions of epileptiform activity are older at seizure onset, often experience complex partial seizures, and have mild or no mental deficits [54]. In some instances, the EEG recordings may be misleading since tubers may interfere in the transmission of underlying electrographic anomalies to the scalp resulting in false-negative surface EEG [76].

Infants with infantile spasms associated with TSC generally present a particular awake interictal EEG characterized by a multifocal asynchronous pattern of spike discharges and irregular slow activity of 2–3 Hz [28]. The pattern often originates from the posterior temporal and occipital cerebral regions. During NREM sleep, there is evidence of increasing epileptiform activities: the multifocal and focal abnormalities tend to generalize and the typical findings of hypsarrhythmia are easily detected (bursts of more synchronous polyspikes and waves separated by sudden voltage attenuation). The pattern changes during REM sleep when the EEG recordings detect a decreasing epileptiform activity, with suppression of generalized discharges and more restricted areas for the epileptiform foci [28]. The interictal EEG abnormal activities are reproducible according to the anatomical regions, tending to persist in serial EEG records.

There are usually severe sleep problems due to sleep-related epileptic events, which are easily shown by polysomnographic recordings, with an increasing number and increased duration of awakenings after sleep onset and reduction of total sleep time and REM sleep time [28].

Ictal EEG recordings show focal discharge of spikes and polyspikes followed by a generalized irregular slow-wave pattern and sudden flattening of background activity in all regions. In some cases, the first spasms (one seizure consists of a series of spasms) may occur with the disappearance of interictal activity throughout the cluster [28].

The electrophysiological pattern detected at onset, with occipitotemporal spikes, tends to persist during the first 2 years, with the same morphology and location, whereas during sleep multifocal abnormalities associated with bursts of bilateral and more synchronous slow spike waves are observed, resembling those seen in Lennox-Gastaut syndrome. At this point detection of the single epileptic focus of origin may be difficult [28].

Cortical Tubers

Neuroimaging

Indeed, epilepsy in TSC is caused by the presence of typical cortical tubers. They can be found in the fetal brain by the 20th week of gestation and can be detected by fetal MRI at the 24th to 26th week of gestation, remaining generally stable in size and appearance proportionally to the rest of the brain in growing children [14, 34]. The tubers are generally identified at the gray-white-matter interface in the supratentorial space, although 8–15 % of patients with TSC develop infratentorial cerebellar lesions [45]. In infancy, on MRI the cortical tubers appear with high intensity on T1-weighted images and with low signal on T2-weighted images compared to the unmyelinated white matter. In childhood and in adult patients, the tubers have low signal on T1-weighted images and are hyperintense on T2-weighted and FLAIR images [45]. In children younger than 7 years, a characteristic cystic change has been described: on FLAIR sequences the tubers show central signal loss with a peripheral high signal intensity. This finding, along with the identification of the *TSC2* mutation, has been reported to be associated with a more aggressive seizure phenotype [19]. Moreover, cystlike tubers in TSC are not static lesions and can exhibit evolving characteristics over time on subsequent MRIs [20]. In the first years of using MRI, two main types of lesions were disclosed by MRI investigations: the first corresponded to smoothly expanded cortical lesions, defined as Pellizzi 1 tubers, and the second showed surface umbilication, defined as Pellizzi 2 tubers, with a central core isointense to CSF [49]. Recently, Gallagher et al. [42] proposed a classification of tuber, along with a spectrum of clinical severity, into three types: (1) Type A tuber are isointense on volumetric T1 images and subtly hyperintense on T2-weighted and fluid-attenuated inversion recovery (FLAIR); (2) type B tubers are hypointense on volumetric T1 images and homogeneously hyperintense on T2-weighted and FLAIR; and (3) type C tubers are hypointense on volumetric T1 images, hyperintense on T2-weighted, and heterogeneous on FLAIR, characterized by a hypointense central region surrounded by a hyperintense rim. Patients with type A tuber dominance have a milder phenotype. Patients with type C tuber dominance have more MRI abnormalities such as subependymal giant cell tumors and are more likely to have an autism spectrum disorder, a history of infantile spasms, and a higher frequency of epileptic seizures compared to patients who have type B tuber dominance, and especially compared to those with a type A dominance. Calcified features are described in half of the cortical tubers and they increase with age and are well detected on CT images or as significant hypointensity on T2-weighted images and gradient echo sequences [43]. Contrast enhancement is present in about 3–4 % of the cases. Because of the reduction of neurons and gliosis and the presence of immature neurons, MR spectroscopy shows a decrease of N-acetylaspartate (NAA) and an increased level of myoinositol, but without any significant difference in the choline (Cho)/Cr ratio [14, 45, 78, 121].

Neuropathology

Cortical tubers are focal abnormalities of cortical architecture, characterized by a proliferation of both glial and dysplastic neurons and a marked disorganization of cortical lamination [23, 45, 80, 81]. Tubers have been considered static lesions, with no acquired malignancy; however, they may appear more prominent over time due to interval myelination and other factors [50].

Macroscopically, the tubers are located at the crest of the cortical gyri and appear as well circumscribed, pale, firm, slightly raised areas of the cortex. More rarely, tubers may be located on the surface of the cerebellar hemispheres. They tend to be confined to a single gyrus or may extend across the adjacent gyri. On cross-sectioning, they have a variable appearance with mushroom-shaped gyri and there is loss of the border between gray and white matter. The surface may be gritty due to calcification, and, in some cases, they undergo cystic degeneration. They vary in number from one to many and in size from microscopic to several centimeters, and have lobar as well as hemispheric distribution. The histological features of tubers were first described by Pellizzi in 1901 [95]. Microscopically, the normal cortical layering is completely lost, with a decreased density of neurons and prominent abnormal cell types such as large dysplastic neurons, giant cells, and bizarrely shaped astrocytes. Examination of the pathological tissue may reveal the presence of activated microglial cells and disruption of blood-brain barrier permeability [10]. The dysmorphic neurons show loss of radial orientation with respect to the pial surface, presenting prominent nucleoli, multiple nuclei, aberrant dendritic arborization, abnormal shape, and accumulation of perikaryal fibrils. The tubers may exhibit cytoskeletal abnormalities with neurofibrillary tangles, argentophilic globules, and granulovacuolar degeneration [23]. The glial element consists in gemistocytic astrocytes with abundant, eosinophilic cytoplasm. The tubers also contain cells of indeterminate neuronal versus glial phenotype with nucleolated nucleus and glassy amphophilic or eosinophilic cytoplasm [45]. The identification of giant bizarre cells is a characteristic feature of cortical tubers in TSC: these cells are similar to the "balloon cells" found in focal cortical dysplasia type 2B and show eccentric nuclei with abundant eosinophilic cytoplasm. These cells can be identified across the thickness of the tuber, distributed along a radial pathway from subcortical white matter or in layer I, and be in a single unit or clumped together in a cluster or chains. Perituberal cortex may have normal cytoarchitecture or may exhibit minor dysplasia or neuronal heterotopias [81]. The background neuropil in the tuber results altered by irregular areas of myelinated fibers and dense fibrillary gliosis, determining the firmness of the tuber [23]. The tubers found in the cerebellum exhibit significant disorganization of cortical layers, with ectopic neurons in the molecular and granule cell layers and white matter; the typical cerebral giant cells as well as calcifications and gliotic degeneration may also be observed [45].

Immunohistochemistry

Several studies have been undertaken to clarify the immunohistochemical features of tubers. The glial cells show a high proportion of glial fibrillary acid protein (GFAP)-positive cells in tubers, not so expressed in the other cerebral lesions (subependymal nodules or SEGA), suggesting that the acquisition of GFAP may occur in association with migration [23, 91]. There is an increased expression of the adhesion molecule CD44, and microglial cells within tubers may express CD68 [45]. Dysmorphic neurons express glutamate transporters such as EAAC1; they exhibit positive immunoreactivity for neurofilament as expression of neuronal differentiation, but these cells may also stain for nestin, vimentin, and other intermediate filaments, indicating that the migration and differentiation processes are disturbed [23, 47]. Giant cells represent a highly heterogeneous population, with some extending microtubule-associated protein 2 (MAP2)-positive dendrites, whereas others extend several small neurofilament-positive processes, suggestive of axons. The immunohistochemical and molecular studies undertaken so far have indicated that the neuronal populations in the tubers may have intrinsic epileptogenicity and actively participate in the generation of a seizure through the release of neurotransmitters or neuromodulators into the adjacent cortex. There is evidence of increased instability of neuronal networks within the epileptogenic tubers, as some authors described, showing a decreased expression pattern of the synaptic vesicle protein 2A, which is the binding site for the antiepileptic drug (AED) levetiracetam [110].

Epileptogenesis

During the last decade there have been several studies to clarify the epileptogenicity in TSC, widening the pathophysiological hypothesis of its onset [50]. There is not a single explanation and the causes must be sought in the different morphological and molecular abnormalities observed in the cortical tubers and the perituberal cortex.

Morphological Features

Cortical tubers originate during fetal development (between 7 and 12 weeks of human gestation) as the result of a primary disorder of neural proliferation [4]. They are generally located at the gray-white-matter border; multiple in number, they are often associated with multiple epileptic foci. Tubers located in the temporal and occipital cerebral lobes, areas of the brain that develop earlier, can become epileptogenic before other cortical lesions in the same patient [81]. Each tuber may differ from the others, even in the same patient, with a wide spectrum of abnormal cell types in different tubers; this might explain the different susceptibility of each tuber to seizure onset and diffusion [34, 50]. According to some authors [19, 41], cystlike cortical tubers may contribute to the more severe epilepsy profile seen in TSC patients with these lesions. Quadrants containing the greatest tuber burden, largest tubers, and calcified tubers were not predictive of regional interictal epileptiform activity.

Numerous morphological features in tubers, as already described in the Neuropathology subsection above, might predispose the patient to the development of seizure: the anomalous cerebral cortical cytoarchitecture, the associated astrocytic proliferation, the presence of calcifications, anomalous vascular anatomy, edema, altered neurotransmitter receptor expression, and the balance between cell proliferation and death all might contribute [50].

The GABA Hypothesis

Epileptogenesis in tubers is supposed to be caused by an imbalance of decreased inhibition, as a consequence of molecular changes in GABA receptors in giant cells and dysplastic neurons, and enhanced excitation, secondary to molecular changes of glutamate receptors in dysplastic neurons [32]. Both inhibitory and excitatory neuronal transmission networks are developmentally regulated. The neurotransmitter gamma-aminobutyric acid (GABA) plays a crucial role in excitatory transmission during early development. It operates primarily via chloride-permeable GABA(A) receptor channels. At an early stage, neurons have a higher intracellular chloride concentration, leading to an efflux of chloride and excitatory actions of GABA in immature neurons. In addition, depolarizing GABA has a strong impact on synaptic plasticity and pathological insults, notably seizures of the immature brain [5]. Later on, damage or loss of inhibitory cortical GABA interneurons is associated with impaired inhibitory control of neocortical pyramidal cells, leading to hyperexcitability and epileptogenesis [111]. The literature report a decreased expression of GABA synthetic enzyme isoform GAD65, vesicular GABA transporter VGAT, and GABA receptor subunits $\alpha1$ and $\alpha2$ in dysplastic neurons of tubers [116]. Moreover, the GABAergic interneurons are particularly vulnerable to cell damage induced by seizures, so that they appear significantly reduced in the early stage of epileptogenesis [81]. There is also evidence of a relationship between neuroactive steroids and seizure susceptibility [31]; in particular, Di Michele et al. [38] reported a reduced ratio between the $3\alpha,5\alpha$- and $3\alpha,5\beta$-tetrahydroprogesterones ($3\alpha_S$-THP), which are positive modulators of $GABA_A$ receptors, and their endogenous functional antagonists $3\beta,5\alpha$- and $3\beta,5\beta$-THP, resulting in reduced sensitivity of $GABA_A$ receptors to GABA and a decreased GABAergic tone.

The Glutamatergic Hypothesis

The GABA signaling is established developmentally before the glutamatergic signaling, but in TSC ionotropic glutamate receptors (iGluRs) also result impaired [106, 116]. In particular, whereas in normal early development the iGluRs are physiologically overexpressed, afterwards there is a progressive reduction. TSC is associated with higher expression of NMDA receptor subunits (subunits NR2B and NR2D), GluR subunits, and AMPA receptor-mediated currents [116, 118]. Dysplastic neurons, giant cells, and dysplastic astroglia in TSC express high levels of pS6 and demonstrate altered GluR subunit composition, resembling that of normal immature neurons and glia [106]. Differences in iGluR expression profiles between dysplastic and nondysplastic epileptic tissue suggest that in human cortical tubers, the *TSC1/TSC2* alteration may alter the developmental regulation of iGluRs and increase the glutamatergic function [86]. The metabotropic glutamate receptors (mGluRs) are also involved in the regulation of the proliferation, differentiation, and survival of neural stem/progenitor cells, as well as in tumor control, playing a role in regulating the extracellular levels of glutamate [17]. Recent studies have demonstrated their possible connection with the hyperexcitability of cells within TSC cortical tubers, resulting in overexpression mainly in dysplastic neurons [8]. Moreover, data from experimental studies have shown a direct link between mGluR activation and the mammalian target of rapamycin (mTOR), which is the main pathway disrupted in TSC [51].

Genetic Influences

TSC1 and *TSC2* mutations have proven to be determinant in the development of structural aberrations in neurons and dendrites. The soma size and dendrite size and density of hippocampal pyramidal cells are perturbed by the loss of a single copy of the *TSC1* gene, which leads to increased AMPA receptor-mediated currents as well [107]. Astrogliosis in the tubers has been connected to mTOR cascade activation in astrocytes (as the result of *TSC1/TSC2* mutations), determining also a specific deficiency in potassium and glutamate uptake of the astrocytes [86, 103].

The Inflammatory Implications

Recently, new insights into cortical tuber epileptogenicity might result from the observation of persistent and complex activation of inflammatory pathways in cortical tubers [9, 11]. In these studies the tubers were characterized by the prominent presence of microglial cells expressing class II antigens (HLA-DR) and, to a lesser extent, the presence of CD68-positive macrophages. There was perivascular and parenchymal T lymphocytes [CD3(+)], with a predominance of CD8(+) T-cytotoxic/suppressor lymphoid cells. Activated microglia and reactive astrocytes expressed IL-1β and its signaling receptor IL-1RI, as well as components of the complement cascade, such as C1q, C3c, and C3d. Albumin extravasation, with uptake in astrocytes, was observed, suggesting that alterations in blood-brain barrier permeability are associated with inflammation in TSC-associated lesions. Intercellular adhesion molecule-1 (ICAM-1), generally activated by inflammation in the cytokine signaling pathway, is increased in tubers but not in the perituberal cortex [77]. However, a clear relationship between the epileptogenicity of cortical tubers and their inflammatory features remains to be clarified.

A Diffuse Cortical Pathology

The concept that epileptogenicity in TSC depends exclusively on the presence of cortical tubers might seem simplistic, considering that surgical removal of the tubers might result in seizure recurrence in about one third of the cases [50]. The epileptogenicity arising from the perituberal regions has been documented by electrocorticography studies and by using AMT-PET (α-[^{11}C]methyl-L-tryptophan) [18, 73, 76]. Actually, there is little information about the morphological features of the perituberal cortex in light of a normal-cortex-sparing policy during surgery. Normal cerebral tissue, as well as the presence of dysplastic cortex, or perituberal gliosis has been described.

As in cases of other malformations of cortical development, there might be a more disseminated distribution of microscopic dysplastic areas, not identifiable on MRI sequences, that cause a wider distribution of the epileptogenic area [50]. In fact, in some cases, interictal epileptiform discharges have been detected from cerebral quadrants without any apparent tuber, suggesting a multifactorial component of epileptogenicity in TSC [41]. Moreover, the case of a tuberless TSC infant associated with intractable epilepsy and developmental delay has recently been reported in the literature [65].

Recently, through the use of the paired transcranial magnetic stimulation protocol (pTMS), an enhanced facilitation of conditioned motor responses following activation of ipsilateral parietal cortex has also been described in TSC, suggesting an amplified cortical connectivity, at least in the parietomotor axonal tract. The existence of pathological corticocortical communication may be determined by the presence of abnormal mechanisms of neuronal excitability control, influencing also the spread of epileptic activity to brain regions distant from the origin of the epileptic focus [36].

Medical Treatment

The probability of developing an epileptic syndrome after a single seizure in TSC patients is extremely high. The prevalence of recurrent seizures in the early phases of cerebral growth may interfere with the development of cortex networks, leading to long-lasting sequelae, namely, cognitive deficits of varying degree, and secondary activation of multiple epileptogenic focus far from the initial onset area, well known as the "kindling" mechanism. Therefore, strong consideration should be given to early treatment with antiepileptic drugs after the first epileptic episode [21]. Considered one of the main dysfunctions responsible for epileptogenesis in TSC, the GABA-mediated synaptic inhibition pathway has been identified as one of the principal medical targets to control seizures. On these grounds, vigabatrin has been considered a first-line treatment for TSC-associated epilepsy. It has been used as an effective antiepileptic drug to reduce infantile spasms in about 50 % of patients, and it has been found most effective in infantile spasms due to tuberous sclerosis (TSC) in which up to 95 % of infants had complete cessation of their spasms [2, 27]. Vigabatrin was synthesized to enhance inhibitory gamma-aminobutyric acidergic (GABAergic) transmission by increasing the synaptic concentration of GABA in the brain via irreversible inhibition of GABA transaminase. Moreover, according to some authors [13], starting vigabatrin at the very onset of seizure, even in cases of partial motor seizures, results in an improved outcome; in particular, in their series no patients who took vigabatrin for focal epilepsy developed infantile spasm. Vigabatrin seems able to stop or prevent diffusion of the paroxysmal activity outside the dysplasia. Its efficacy is usually observed within a week, showing better results with focal seizures originating from parieto-occipital lobes [31].

Recent studies in the pediatric population showed that vigabatrin administration is associated with reversible and asymptomatic diffusion abnormalities, such as myelin edema lesions, in globi pallidi, thalami, brainstem, and dentate nuclei. More frequent in younger infants, these abnormalities have been reported to be transient and dose-dependent, with the majority resolving spontaneously, even without discontinuing vigabatrin [79, 109]. Psychotic disorders or hallucinations have rarely occurred [117]. Actually, the main concern with taking vigabatrin therapy is the reported late occurrence of visual-field defects in up to 50 % of patients who underwent it; it depends on the age of the patient and the extent of exposure to vigabatrin. The earliest finding of the first abnormal field examination in adults was reported to be after 9 months of treatment, with a mean duration of vigabatrin exposure of 4.8 years, whereas in children, the earliest onset was reported to be after 11 months, with a mean time to onset of 5.5 years [117]. Considering that the effectiveness of vigabatrin can be detected within 12 weeks of initiating therapy, and in some cases even after 1–2 doses [81], the risk of developing a peripheral visual field deficit with short-term exposure seems to be low. Nevertheless, if the treatment is continued, periodic monitoring for the peripheral visual field deficit is necessary [117].

The responsiveness of seizure in TSC patients to vigabatrin does not seem completely related to the known pathophysiology of epilepsy. Indeed, treatment with other anticonvulsants, including other drugs that interfere with the GABA system, did not result in good seizure control [50]. Medical treatment can be switched with other antiepileptic drugs such as topiramate, which presents multiple mechanisms of action, or combination therapy with carbamazepine, valproate, and zonisamide can be used [13]. Recently, the combination of levetiracetam with GABAergic agonists or valproate and lamotrigine has proved to have some efficacy [81]. Indeed, there is no clear evidence of the superiority of one drug over the other and the final choice will eventually depend on availability, tolerability, and cost [23].

The ketogenic diet has proved to be as efficacious in TSC patients as in other refractory epilepsy patients [67]. In other respects, data on confirmed efficacy of the ketogenic diet in TSC epilepsy are still lacking, despite numerous reported retrospective and prospective studies [23]. It is supposed to have a differential sensitivity due to mechanistic implications. Some recent reports described the presence of overexpressed multidrug-resistant proteins MDR-1 and MRP-1 as well as a breast cancer-resistant protein, over different cellular components of resected tubers, including giant cells, dysplastic neurons, microglia, and astrocytes [69].

Future Perspectives: Rapamycin

The discovery of the mTOR pathway upregulation in TSC patients and its implications in tumorigenesis has introduced new possibilities for treatment strategies [32, 89].

Rapamycin, also known as sirolimus, was discovered in 1965 from soil samples on Easter Island and was called Rapa Nui by the indigenous population. Approved by the US Food and Drug Administration in the 1999 for the prophylaxis of organ rejection, it has powerful antiproliferative and immunosuppressant activity [32].

Its exact mechanism of action is still the subject of research; however, there have been several in vitro and in vivo studies which suggested that rapamycin might be effective in the treatment of various manifestations of TSC, since it can normalize the mTOR pathway dysregulated in the cells that lack TSC1 or TSC2.

Sirolimus mediates protein synthesis stimulated by brain-derived neurotrophic factors and presents neurophysiologic effects through direct association with the FK506 binding protein (FKBP12) [86]. The rapamycin/FKBP12 complex binds with high affinity to mTOR. Its activity causes depression of specific protein phosphatases, which leads to dephosphorylation of mTOR downstream effectors such as S6K1 and 4E-BP1, thus increasing levels of unphosphorylated S6K which causes inhibition of translation and cell cycle arrest [85].

Moreover, rapamycin has been proven to have an effect on VEGF production, reducing the angiogenetic process in the vascular tumors typical of TSC, including cutaneous angiofibromas and lymphangioleiomyomatosis (LAM). Recent clinical trials have demonstrated the reduction (in some cases transitory) of tumor volume in cases of renal angiomyolipomas, subependymal giant cell tumors (SEGAs), and angiofibromas, and improved pulmonary function in sporadic LAM [6, 48, 82].

The efficacy of rapamycin in seizure control and in reversing mental retardation has been tested in mouse models [125]. Early treatment with rapamycin prevented the development of epilepsy and premature death that were observed in vehicle-treated Tsc1(GFAP)CKO mice, whereas late treatment with rapamycin suppressed seizures and prolonged survival in Tsc1(GFAP)CKO mice that had already developed epilepsy. So far, only sporadic cases in the literature reported a dramatic reduction in seizure frequency in human beings [84].

Epilepsy Surgery

Despite complicated antiepileptic drug combinations and even after initial response to medical therapy, about two thirds of epilepsy patients (62.5 % according to Chu-Shore et al. [21]) are refractory to medication and may be possible candidates for epilepsy surgery. A general principle of epilepsy surgery is that its success depends on identifying the exact area of origin of seizures and defining its topographic edges and functional relationship with eloquent areas to assess the safety and risks of resection [12]. Therefore, finding the correspondence between clinical, electrophysiological, and radiological data is the goal of the preoperative evaluation. However, the patients affected by TSC have the worst characteristics for successful epilepsy surgery: extratemporal, multifocal, bilateral, and often overlapping eloquent areas. Moreover, the intracranial electrode monitoring may be limited by the presence of secondary epileptogenic foci that may be unmasked by the excision of the primary focus [114]. Thus, it remains challenging to distinguish epileptogenic from nonepileptogenic tubers in TSC patients. In some cases, seizures can start independently from different tubers or other tubers may be activated secondarily after the specific onset tuber in such a rapid way that the results may be indistinguishable. In other cases, the epileptic focus does not coincide with a tuber and there is widespread epileptogenicity not limited to the structural abnormalities seen on MRI [53].

Presurgical Workup

The preoperative evaluation of patients affected by epilepsy related to TSC disease starts with taking a detailed family, birth, and personal history. It also consists of physical and neurological examinations, neuropsychiatric testing, routine MRI [including diffusion-weighted MRI (DWI) and proton magnetic resonance spectroscopy (MRS)] and CT scans, and electrophysiological studies, including interictal EEG and prolonged video-EEG monitoring [12, 99]. To achieve better presurgery localization, there is increasing widespread use of complementary noninvasive functional mapping studies, namely, magnetoencephalography (MEG), positron emission tomography (PET), and ictal and interictal single-photon emission computed tomography (SPECT), which have demonstrated substantial promise [12, 31]. On the other hand, a final attempt to identify precisely the epileptogenic focus is made by using invasive electrophysiological monitoring with electrocorticography and invasive video EEG [12, 55, 76, 114].

Interictal-Ictal EEG

Scalp EEG is generally the first attempt to obtain important clues on the focal nature of seizure onset, but it is not good at detecting the epileptogenic focus for surgical planning [99]. According to some authors, the correspondence of cortical tubers and electroencephalographic foci is visible in less than 50 % of cases [35], demonstrating the limited spatial resolution of scalp interictal EEG. However, in 90 % of patients with a long history of epilepsy and mild developmental delay, there is at least one region of consistent interictal epileptiform activity that is generally associated with complex partial seizures [54]. The long-term ictal video-EEG monitoring is mandatory. Nevertheless, analysis of the ictal EEG has lagged behind that of the interictal spikes because of the noise ratio, particularly for movements and EMG artifacts induced by the ictal phenomenon and due to the dynamic character of the epileptic activity which diffuses to various brain regions. Independent component analysis of ictal EEG events and source analysis methods are effective tools to establish the connection between epileptic scalp activity and the cortical tubers [70]. In 79 % of cases there is concordance between the dominant and consistent interictal focus and the ictal onset zone [114]. The short time lag estimation is also becoming a valuable tool to identify the lateralized onset of apparently bilateral discharges [31, 99].

MEG/MSI

Magnetoencephalography (MEG) is a useful tool for identifying the epileptogenic tuber in patients with focal seizures [12]. The fusion of electroencephalographic and magnetoencephalographic data improves the functional localization; they both provide complementary information, with the scalp EEG detecting tangential and radial sources and the MEG measuring exclusively the tangential sources [99]. Magnetic source imaging (MSI) is a technique that fuses the MEG-originated current dipole localizations on three-dimensional references, with multiplanar images from MRI [119]. This technique provides good results in localizing the epileptogenic focus in about 80 % of a series of patients with TSC, with a strict correlation between removal of the MSI dipole cluster and postoperative seizure freedom [120]. Synthetic aperture magnetometry (SAM) is a recently developed adaptive spatial filtering algorithm for MEG that provides automated temporal detection of spike sources by using the excess kurtosis value (steepness of an epileptic spike in the virtual sensor-SAM kurtosis algorithm), with some advantages over the equivalent current dipole (ECD) model [105]. The combination of the SAM kurtosis algorithm and ECD analyses allowed the localization of complex epileptic zones in patients with multiple cortical tubers, obtaining seizure freedom in six of eight patients operated on [105].

PET

Positron emission tomography (PET) shows the metabolism of radiolabeled tracers. Its coregistration with morphological images from MRI allows the localization of areas with altered substrate metabolism, often correlated with ictal onset zones [12]. The most used tracers, recently introduced as more specific in identifying epileptogenic tubers, are fluorodeoxyglucose (FDG-PET) and 11-C-methyl-L-tryptophan, a tracer for serotonin synthesis and tryptophan metabolism via the kynurenine pathway (AMT-PET). FDG-PET coregistered with MRI shows a decreased interictal glucose metabolism on active tubers, with a postoperative seizure freedom rate of 67 % compared with 68 % achieved with the invasive intracranial recording approach [120]. AMT-PET has recently demonstrated a high uptake of radioactive ligands, distinguishing between epileptogenic and electrically silent tubers and establishing that an uptake of 1.0 or more is associated with improved outcome after surgery [23, 31]. AMT-PET proved to be more effective in helping with proper positioning of subdural electrodes, even when coregistration of FDG-PET and MRI failed to provide adequate localizing data [31].

SPECT

Ictal and interictal single-photon emission computed tomography (SPECT) has been widely used in detecting the epileptogenic focus in epilepsy patients, showing focal hyperperfusion during seizure in the region of the ictal onset. Ictal SPECT has demonstrated a sensitivity similar to that of FDG-PET, improved by the SISCOM technique (Subtraction Ictal SPECT CO-registered to MRI), by detecting regional differences between interictal and ictal perfusion [12]. It has been shown that pre-operative SISCOM improves information for invasive electrode placement in children with multiple lesions, as does TSC [1].

EEG-fMRI

Simultaneous EEG and functional MRI (3-T) has been introduced to evaluate the epileptogenic networks in the brains of patients with TSC, combining the temporal resolution of the EEG with the spatial resolution of a high-field MRI. Already used to define the irritative focus in sedated children with good results [53], it is a relatively recent noninvasive tool that allows the detection of areas with Blood Oxygenation Level-Dependent (BOLD) signal changes correlated with the interictal epileptic discharges [53]. The study conducted by Jacobs et al. [53] suggested the existence of extended epileptogenic networks, exceeding those described in PET and SPECT studies; they were able to identify specific interictally active tubers, demonstrating that BOLD changes were limited to restricted areas of the tuber, especially to one side or at the edge of the tuber, and in some cases in perilesional areas, even exclusively. The BOLD response was observed in the area corresponding to the interictal epileptic discharges in 77 % of cases, but it also was detected in other regions of the brain, distant from the epileptic discharge, suggesting the presence of potential irritative zones contributing to the spread or generation of epilepsy. Unexpectedly, Jacobs et al. [53] found a BOLD response in a subependymal astrocytoma, supporting the hypothesis that since subependymal astrocytomas derive from stem cells and consist of proliferating neuronal and glial cells, they may be part of the epileptogenic network. Indeed, the surgical excision of a SEGA often may be followed by a reduction or the transient disappearance of seizures. However, other factors could account for the phenomenon, including the characteristic of the surgical approach (partial callosotomy in case of interhemispheric approach) or surgically induced reduction of the associated obstructive hydrocephalus [39].

Invasive Monitoring

Invasive monitoring with subdural electrodes is indicated when the video-EEG examination fails to determine a precise relationship between the ictal onset area and the anatomical lesions detected on MR images. The use of invasive video EEG has often been advocated in cases where there is discordant noninvasive information, multifocal pathology, ictal onset in proximity to eloquent areas, and lesions with chronic epilepsy with ictal onset from the perituberal cortex [12]. Madhavan et al. [74] proposed a three-stage invasive approach: first, implantation of subdural electrodes and subsequent resection of the ictal onset zone; second, the subdural electrodes are reimplanted over the resection area and surrounding zone to identify any residual seizure foci to be removed by a second resection. In selected patients with multifocal and bilateral tuber seizure foci, aggressive bilateral invasive monitoring has been adopted [114]. This multistage approach has allowed the identification of primary and secondary epileptogenic foci in patients with multiple tubers, obtaining a seizure freedom rate of about 65 % at a 2-year follow-up. According to the authors promoting this multistage approach [12], it has some disadvantages, namely, the need for additional surgery and the subsequent increased cost, length of hospital stay, and potential morbidity. However, even though an alternative one- or two-stage resection of dominant tuber/seizure focus can be proposed, considering further surgery only if seizures persist, the authors believe that it is easier to carry out the complete resection in a single hospital stay rather than bring back the patient and the family later on [12]. Advanced MEG tools and simultaneous EEG and fMRI can precisely define the ictal onset zone detected by invasive electrodes [81].

Epileptogenic tubers may arise in eloquent cerebral zones, causing serious concern for postoperative neurological morbidity. Actually, whereas it has been reported that other epileptogenic lesions such as focal cortical dysplasia or low-grade gliomas maintain functional activity, no clear data have been reported on the functional content of cortical tubers [83]. Considering that awake surgery might be extremely difficult in patients affected by TSC, who generally present with mental delay and behavioral problems or, especially lately, are more often very young children, some authors [83] have used intraoperative and extraoperative subdural electrode recordings to define the epileptogenic cortex and map functional cortical areas and obtained good seizure control and low neurological morbidity. On these grounds, there is supposed to be a reorganization of functional cortex or simply no functional cortex in tubers arising in rolandic or perirolandic cortex.

The increasingly frequent offer of surgery for the treatment of drug-resistant epilepsy and the need to localize a unique and resectable epileptic zone increase the use of other types of invasive recordings such as stereoelectroencephalography

(SEEG). In SEEG, the EEG recording is obtained from intracerebral, stereotactically placed, platinum-iridium, semiflexible, multicontact electrodes, the number of which varies according to the characteristics of the patient. Compared with subdural grids or strips, which cover a larger but more superficial cortical surface, SEEG offers the advantage of being able to completely investigate the pathway between the cortex and the deep cerebral structures with a less invasive surgical operation together with the possibility of performing intracerebral electric stimulation; its main limit is the relatively small volume of tissue recorded by each electrode.

SEEG may be indicated for children requiring resective surgery (except for hemispherectomy) when the correlations among anatomical, clinical, and electrophysiological data are incoherent. Tuberous sclerosis is sporadically mentioned as an indication for SEEG in large series compared with focal cortical dysplasia or "isolated" pediatric brain tumors [25, 26]. This is probably because of the relative rarity of TSC, compared with other causes of seizures, and/or because of the acceptable anatomo-clinico-electric correlation in some cases. Moreover, the presence of several associated brain lesions may prevent the insertion of an adequate number of electrodes, at least in some instances. At the same time, the concomitance of multiple lesions as a possible source of epilepsy, scattered within a hemisphere, favors the use of the subdural grid for invasive monitoring. However, SEEG may have an important role in selected cases of TSC, namely, when there is clinical and EEG evidence of localized ictal onset in spite of bilateral and multifocal tubers. SEEG may also be useful when tubers are close to eloquent areas: in this case, SEEG allows one to analyse and understand the functional mapping that is required to assess the surgical risks and the prognosis of the surgical resection on epilepsy.

Surgical Procedures

Refractory epilepsy occurs in approximately two thirds of epilepsy patients, consequently requiring consideration of nonmedical treatment. Initially introduced by Achslog J in 1964 [55], during the last five decades surgery has been widely considered for the treatment of refractory epilepsy associated with tuberous sclerosis. Surgical options for patients with TSC affected by intractable epilepsy include resection of the epileptogenic cortical area, corpus callosotomy, and vagal nerve stimulation [23, 99].

Resective Surgery

Surgical excision of a single cortical tuber, localized in noneloquent areas and coinciding with EEG evidence of ictal onset, has the best chance to obtain total seizure control. However, this is not the most frequent condition a neurosurgeon may deal with. As mentioned above, patients with TSC and epilepsy often have multiple cortical tubers, generally in both hemispheres. In cases of multiple tubers, seizures may arise from one of them, which may appear to be the largest, but not always. In these

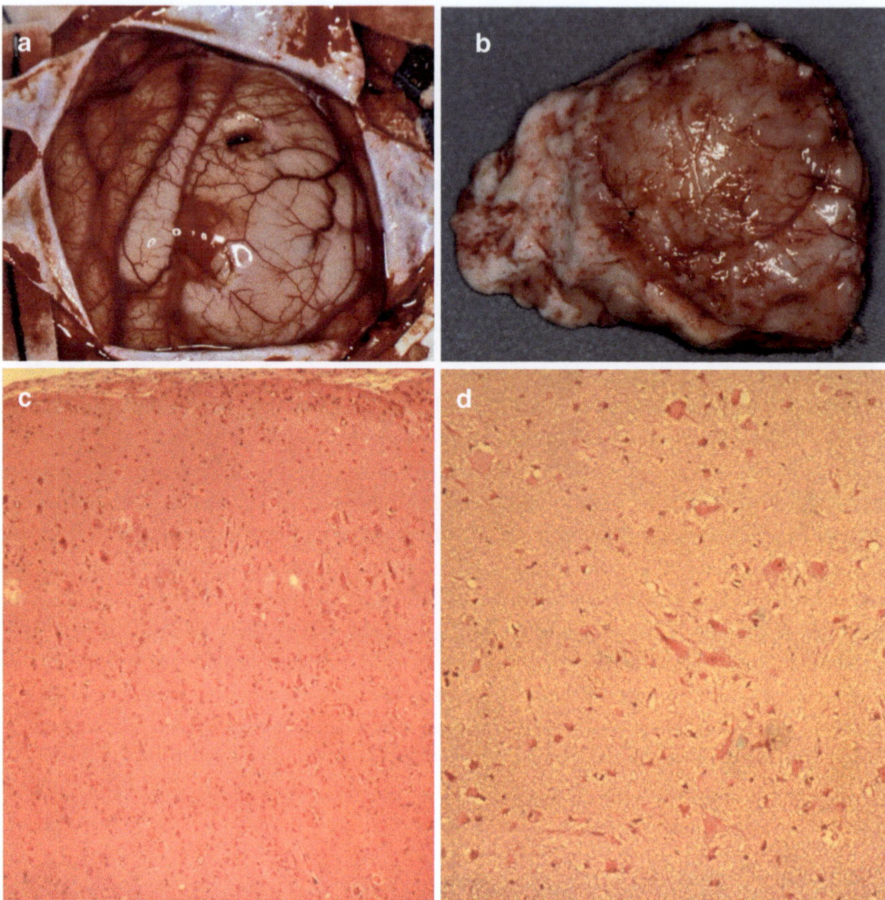

Fig. 2 (**a, b**) Macroscopic appearance of a cortical tuber before (**a**) and after (**b**) the surgical resection. The brain cortex is pale and shows an increased thickness, the gyri are flattened. (**c, d**) Microscopic appearance of the same specimen. Note the absence of the normal cortical layering and the presence of several dysplastic giant neurons and abnormal astrocytes

cases, at the time of surgery, finding the exact tuber that was identified preoperatively as epileptogenic may be difficult when observing only the surface of the brain [23]. Intraoperative aides that can be used are frameless stereotaxy, neuronavigation, and ultrasound. Intraoperative electrocorticography is often advocated during surgery, even when the tuber is obvious. It may confirm the presence of abnormal EEG activity arising from the surface of the tuber and it may also define the borders of the epileptogenic area, which may involve the perituberal region in apparently normal cortex. In this regard, some authors [74, 83, 108] believe that perituberal cortex should be removed as well, because the epileptogenicity may derive from the perturbation or abnormal development of the surrounding cortex rather than from the tuber itself.

Macroscopically the tuber appears as a slightly expanded gyrus, firm to the touch (Fig. 2). Once identified, it is resected by going around its boundaries and dissecting

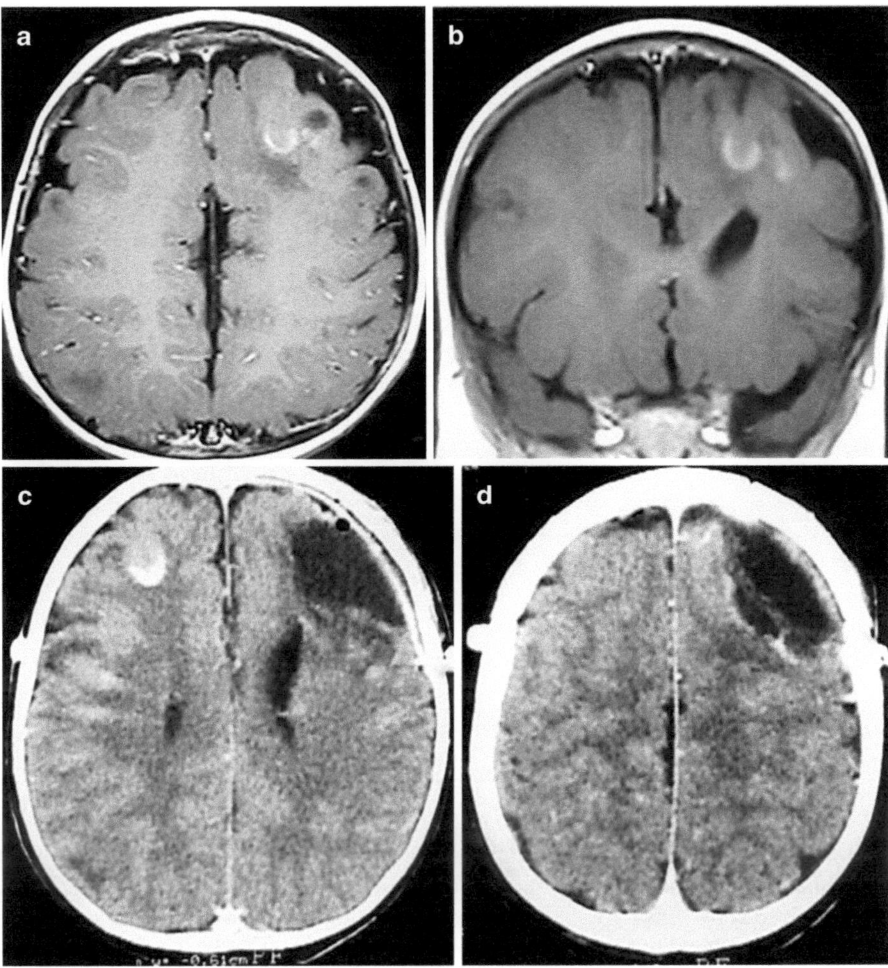

Fig. 3 (**a**) Postcontrast axial T1-weighted and (**b**) coronal T1-weighted MR images showing a left frontal tuber lesion in a TSC patient. (**c**, **d**) Postsurgical CT scans of the same patient

it from the surrounding normal cortex; a gyral cleavage plane may be observed, facilitating the procedure. Large tubers may extend over multiple gyri and frequently crossing veins are encountered. According to some authors, the veins can be easily dissected away from the tuber, which eventually can be totally removed [23] (Fig. 3).

The contiguity or coincidence of the epileptogenic tuber with eloquent areas may be challenging in resective surgery. In this case, some authors recommend a multiple subpial transection in the involved eloquent areas [23, 99], and other authors use intraoperative electrocortical monitoring which has allowed good seizure control and low neurological morbidity in a recent series [83].

Table 2 Seizure freedom after epilepsy surgery in TSC patients from selected series in the last 10 years

Authors	Number of cases	Epilepsy outcome
Leiphart et al. [71]	14	7/14 Engel I (50 %)
Ohta et al. [88]	1	0
Bittar et al. [7]	1	0
Karenfort et al. [63]	8	3/8 Engel I (37 %)
Romanelli et al. [98]	2	1/2 Engel I (50 %)
Vigliano et al. [113]	4	2/4 Engel I (50 %)
Kossoff et al. [66]	2	2/2 Engel I (100 %)
Mackay et al. [72]	7	3/7 Engel I (43 %)
O'Connor et al. [87]	2	1/2 Engel I (50 %)
Asano et al. [3]	8	6/8 Engel I (75 %)
Kagawa et al. [62]	17	12/17 Engel I (71 %)
Lachhwani et al. [68]	17	15/17 Engel I (89 %)
Connolly et al. [23]	7	2/7 Engel I (28.5 %)
Madhavan et al. [74] (multicentric study)	70	37/70 Engel I (53 %)
Leal et al. [70]	3	3/3 Engel I (100 %)
Teutonico et al. [108]	11	3/11 Engel I (27 %)
Bollo et al. [12]	45	30/45 Engel I (67 %)
Major et al. [76]	3	1/3 Engel I (33 %)
Sugiyama et al. [105]	8	6/8 Engel I (75 %)
Moshel et al. [83]	15	9/15 Engel I (60 %)
van der Heide et al. [112]	6	3/6 Engel I (50 %)
Wu et al. [120]	18	12/18 Engel I (67 %)
Kassiri et al. [64]	11	10/11 Engel I (90.9 %)

Lesionectomy or tuberectomy is even more complicated in the setting of multiple and bilateral electric abnormalities detected on electrophysiological recordings. As described above, invasive monitoring with subdural grids can be used, at least when seizures can be lateralized to one hemisphere, when PET or SPECT fail to identify a specific epileptogenic tuber [23]. This allows the identification of the single or multiple epileptogenic tubers to be resected. Bilateral subdural electrocorticography has recently been introduced considering possible bilateral tuberectomies safe and effective procedures, according to the three-stage approach described previously [12, 74].

Indeed, based on these invasive approaches, the indications for surgery are ever widening to include patients with poor quality of life who traditionally would have not met the surgical criteria: in particular, very young patients, who generally present with catastrophic epileptic syndrome associated with developmental delay and regression and patients with multiple potentially epileptogenic cortical tubers [12]. These aggressive approaches are associated with significant control of epilepsy as well as improved quality of life for the patient and the family [100].

Despite considerable variation among the studies reported in the literature, including different clinical characteristics of the patients, namely, age at epilepsy onset or age at surgery, or various presurgical techniques and surgical procedures adopted, the overall results of selected series have shown that epilepsy surgery is successful in patients with drug-resistant epilepsy and TSC (Table 2) [55, 81].

According to the systematic review by Jansen et al. [55], seizure freedom was achieved in 57 % and seizure frequency improved by 90 % in another 18 % of patients; thus, there was good seizure control in 75 % of the cases. The seizure freedom rate significantly improved over the last 5 years, leading to 63 % of Engel class I status, probably due to the recent technical advances in the localization of the epileptogenic zone [81]. Indeed, the best seizure control was obtained when a single epileptogenic tuber was individuated and removed. On the other hand, risks factors for surgical failure were tonic seizures, moderate or severe intellectual deficit, and multifocal SPECT abnormalities and MEG dipole clusters, which were reported in only few studies [46, 55, 81]. According to other authors [74], poor seizure freedom outcome is associated with early age of seizure onset, history of infantile spasms, and multifocal interictal activity. Epileptic activation of additional tubers over a life span cannot be forecasted but may lead to reoperation and multi-stage surgery.

Corpus Callosotomy

Corpus callosotomy has been suggested especially for those children with drop attacks as the main disabling seizure type [23]. It is considered a palliative procedure, generally performed with the aim of breaking off seizure generalization in catastrophic epileptic conditions. These patients, in fact, have a generally poor quality of life with severe developmental delay, so complete disconnection of the corpus callosum is not a major concern with respect to the effect of subsequent disconnection syndrome. After this procedure, the primary epileptic focus, which generally persists, can be identified easier, allowing a possible second operation for resection of the epileptogenic tuber [23].

Vagal Nerve Stimulation (VNS)

Vagal nerve implantation is an adjunctive treatment for refractory epilepsies and was introduced after approval by the US Drug and Food Administration in 1997 [23, 122]. In the literature, a few small series of patients with intractable epilepsy associated with TSC have been reported [40, 75, 90, 122], with VNS proving to be a valuable aid when resective surgery is not indicated. According to these studies, a significant reduction of seizure frequency is obtained with VNS in about 70 % of cases and sporadic cases of seizure freedom after VNS have been described [122]. The improvement in seizure control seems to increase with time and to persist at long-term follow-up, particularly for children implanted under 6 years of age [122]. Some authors advocate the use of vagal nerve implantation as soon as possible in selected patients to achieve behavioral and neuropsychological improvements and a better quality of life [81]. There is also evidence that VNS may be effective in improving cognitive deficits independent of seizure activity [81, 122]. Due to the heterogeneity of the populations studied, there are no clear relationships between device efficacy and the clinical characteristics of patients, including gender, age at seizure onset, age at implantation, type of genetic mutation, duration of VNS treatment, infantile spasm, or autism features [40]. Although the precise mechanism of action of vagal nerve stimulation is still unknown, there seems to be a direct effect of reducing cortical excitability by interfering with the $GABA_A$ receptor density [122]. Moreover, the effectiveness of VNS in seizure control appeared greater when the results were compared with those of patients without TSC [40].

Cognitive and Behavioral Aspects

Tuberous sclerosis complex is associated with high rates of cognitive impairment, from mild difficulties in definite areas of cognition to profound mental retardation, and pervasive developmental disorder, namely, autism [37, 52, 58, 96, 123, 124]. Initially reported as part of the classic diagnostic triad for TSC, neither epilepsy nor mental retardation has remained in the list of diagnostic characteristics because of their lack of specificity for the disorder [96]. Moreover, recent studies have documented an incidence of global cognitive impairment in no more than 44–60 % of TSC cases [52, 96, 123]. Tuberous sclerosis is detected in about 1–2 % of people with mental illness. However, improved clinical testing has led to the identification of various specific behavioral and cognitive difficulties in TSC patients who do not present global cognitive impairment. These neuropsychiatric manifestations are of great concern to families and influence dramatically the quality of daily life and disrupt educational and occupational progress [37]. Refractory epilepsy is supposed to worsen preexisting cognitive and behavioral impairment, not responsible just for its occurrence and severity.

Cognitive Impairment

According to recent population-based studies [59], there is a bimodal distribution of the IQ scores of TSC patients: 55 % of subjects were within the normal range (IQ > 80) and 44 % had an IQ score of <70, in the majority of cases with severe to profound mental disabilities (IQ < 21). Those patients in the normal range of global intellectual abilities had a mean IQ 12 points lower than their unaffected siblings, even in the absence of epilepsy history. Intellectual deficits are described by 1 year of age and tend to be stable and persistent [37]. The most compromised TSC children often have arrested development and do not show developmental progress over time. On the other hand, the majority of TSC children will progress in their developmental stages over time, albeit at a slower rate and lower level than their unaffected siblings [96].

Cognitive impairment in TSC has a multifactorial etiopathogenesis. A molecular genetic basis has been described because patients with *TSC2* mutations are more likely to be mentally retarded; however, in reality the genotype accounts for a small fraction of the variation in neurological symptoms [56]. The association between different *TSC1* and *TSC2* mutations and the neurological and cognitive phenotypes was analyzed by James et al. [57], who showed that patients with *TSC2* mutation have an earlier age at seizure onset, a lower mean cognition index, more tubers, and a greater TBP (tuber/brain proportion) than those with *TSC1* mutation. Patients with *TSC2* mutation have more frequent cognitive impairments but they are not more severe than those of patients with *TSC1* mutation. Sporadic mutations were associated with an earlier age at seizure onset and a lower cognition index than familial cases.

The number of tubers has been indicated as a determining factor of increased risk for mental retardation [52], especially when considering that more cortical tubers are related to early-onset epilepsy which negatively influences cognition. However, some have reported that patients with small numbers of tubers may have a worse cognitive outcome than those with multiple lesions [61]. Intellectual impairment is increasingly reported in patients with bilateral tubers than in those with unilateral lesions [124]. According to some authors [57], the proportion of the total brain volume occupied by tubers (tuber/brain proportion, TBP) is a better predictor of cognitive function than the number of tubers, although patients with normal intelligence and large TBP have also been described.

Nevertheless, there is general agreement that the most predictive factor of cognitive impairment is the age of seizure onset. Data from the literature do not report a definite relationship between cognitive delay and the presence of infantile spasms, even though there is an increasing tendency to consider that cessation of infantile spasms leads to improvement in cognitive development [61].

Learning difficulties may also be detected in TSC patients, even in children with normal global intellectual abilities [96]. Data from the literature report a high risk of very specific neuropsychological deficits in attentional-executive skills in TSC patients, even in the absence of global intellectual disorders or a psychiatric diagnosis [96].

Behavioural Sequelae

About half of the patients with TSC have some behavioral difficulties during development, displaying more frequently classic infantile autism, autism spectrum disorder [30, 58] and attention-deficit hyperactivity disorder (ADHD) and related disorders [96].

During adolescence and into adulthood, a great number of patients develop severe affective symptoms, namely, anxiety or depressed mood.

Another common behavioral manifestation is sleep disorder, including night waking, waking early, seizure-related sleep problems, and excessive daytime sleepiness, with reduced rapid-eye-movement sleep, sleep instability, and fragmentation with frequent awakenings [29]. Sleep disorders are supposed to be related mainly o sleep-related events.

In addition, seizures and EEG abnormalities (in particular, temporal lobe epileptic discharges) during early development seem to have a negative impact on the development of those brain systems that underlie social intelligence and other cognitive skills, possibly inducing the autistic spectrum disorder [30, 33].

Genetic factors related to the known mutations are supposed to influence the neurocognitive abnormalities, even though a strict correlation between the genotype and the phenotype has not been demonstrated until now, suggesting that other genetic, epigenetic, and environmental factors modify the severity of behavioral disorders, in particular, the autism [33].

Surgery and pharmacological antiepileptic treatments may improve cognitive and behavioral disorders, interfering with the negative effects of early epilepsy, but a normal cognitive outcome for children affected by TSC cannot be guaranteed, and the children may require intensive behavioral intervention.

Conclusion Remarks

TSC continues to a get a great deal of attention in the scientific community because of the involvement of multiple organs and the challenges related to the follow-up and treatment of the affected patients. Such interest is also indicated by base research which provides much information on TSC genes (more than 350 mutations detected so far) and their function (e.g., relationship with the mTOR signalling cascade).

One of the most intriguing and challenging aspects of TSC is the occurrence of correlated epileptic seizures such that many efforts are currently devoted to assessing its genesis and characteristics and to improve its treatment. We summarize the main advances on the knowledge of TSC as follows:

- Seizures are the most common neurological symptom of TSC, involving more than 80 % of TSC patients. They are prevalent during infancy and childhood but they also can start during adulthood. Spasms represent the most common type of seizure. Patients with a mutated *TSC2* gene are significantly more prone to develop epilepsy than those with *TSC1* gene mutation;
- *TSC2* mutation is also associated with a more aggressive seizure phenotype and with tubers with a cystlike appearance. On MRI, such tubers are self-changing lesions that are usually detected in small children;
- According to MRI appearance, tubers may be classified into three types (A, B, C), each with different radiological characteristics and a different prognosis (type C has the worst prognosis because of the frequent occurrence of associated lesions such as SEGA, and associated disorders such as infantile spasms and autism);

- Tubers continue to be thought to play an active role in epileptogenesis. This hypothesis is based on several data: (1) imbalance between inhibitory (reduction of GABA isoforms, GABA receptors, and vesicular transporter) and excitatory transmission (increased glutamatergic function with overexpression of NMDA receptors and dysregulation of iGluRs) in the tuberal dysplastic neurons, (2) release of neurotransmitters altering the activity of the perituberal cortex, and (3) induction of possible perituberal inflammatory reaction;
- Seizures persist in one third of cases after removal of tubers and they can even occur in the rare "tuberless" TSC. This indicates that the perituberal cortex and other associated lesions exert an epileptogenic action as well. The mechanisms of such an action are being investigated; an abnormal corticocortical connectivity has been recently postulated as one mechanism;
- The medical treatment of TSC epilepsy relies on vigabatrin and/or a combination of antiepileptic drugs and/or a ketogenic diet. Encouraging preliminary results are being obtained with rapamycin according to both in vitro and in vivo studies. Actually, rapamycin can normalize the mTOR pathway (which is upregulated in TSC);
- Potentially, about one third of TSC patients are candidates for surgery because of drug-resistant seizures. However, the frequent occurrence of extratemporal epilepsy with multifocal/bilateral foci may represent an important limit to surgical indication. Therefore, for proper patient selection, the "traditional" preoperative workup (MRI, surface video EEG, SPECT) frequently needs to be complemented with more recently developed examinations (functional MRI, invasive EEG monitoring, magnetoencephalography, PET);
- Lesionectomy or tuberectomy currently make more than 60 % of patients seizure-free (especially if guided by intraoperative electrocortical monitoring). Disappointing results are obtained in the cases with multiple interictal foci and infantile spasms. Callosotomy and vagal nerve stimulation maintain a palliative role;
- Cognitive and behavioral impairments are either disease-related (molecular alterations resulting from *TSC1* and two mutations) and epilepsy-related (drug resistance). About one half of TSC patients have an IQ below the normal range, with severe cognitive retardation in most of them.

References

1. Ahnlide JA, Rosén I, Lindén-Mickelsson Tech P, Källén K (2007) Does SISCOM contribute to favorable seizure outcome after epilepsy surgery? Epilepsia 48(3):579–588
2. Ando N, Fujimoto S, Ishikawa T, Kobayashi S, Hattori A, Ito T, Togari H (2010) Effectiveness of vigabatrin in west syndrome associated with tuberous sclerosis. No To Hattatsu 42(6):444–448
3. Asano E, Juhász C, Shah A, Muzik O, Chugani DC, Shah J, Sood S, Chugani HT (2005) Origin and propagation of epileptic spasms delineated on electrocorticography. Epilepsia 46(7): 1086–1097

4. Barkovich AJ, Kuzniecky RI, Jackson GD, Guerrini R, Dobyns WB (2005) A developmental and genetic classification for malformations of cortical development. Neurology 65(12):1873–1887

5. Ben-Ari Y, Gaiarsa JL, Tyzio R, Khazipov R (2007) GABA: a pioneer transmitter that excites immature neurons and generates primitive oscillations. Physiol Rev 87(4):1215–1284

6. Bissler JJ, McCormack FX, Young LR, Elwing JM, Chuck G, Leonard JM, Schmithorst VJ, Laor T, Brody AS, Bean J, Salisbury S, Franz DN (2008) Sirolimus for angiomyolipoma in tuberous sclerosis complex or lymphangioleiomyomatosis. N Engl J Med 358(2):140–151

7. Bittar RG, Rosenfeld JV, Klug GL, Hopkins IJ, Harvey AS (2002) Resective surgery in infants and young children with intractable epilepsy. J Clin Neurosci 9(2):142–146

8. Boer K, Troost D, Timmermans W, Gorter JA, Spliet WG, Nellist M, Jansen F, Aronica E (2008) Cellular localization of metabotropic glutamate receptors in cortical tubers and subependymal giant cell tumors of tuberous sclerosis complex. Neuroscience 156(1):203–215

9. Boer K, Jansen F, Nellist M, Redeker S, van den Ouweland AM, Spliet WG, van Nieuwenhuizen O, Troost D, Crino PB, Aronica E (2008) Inflammatory processes in cortical tubers and subependymal giant cell tumors of tuberous sclerosis complex. Epilepsy Res 78(1):7–21

10. Boer K, Troost D, Jansen F, Nellist M, van den Ouweland AM, Geurts JJ, Spliet WG, Crino P, Aronica E (2008) Clinicopathological and immunohistochemical findings in an autopsy case of tuberous sclerosis complex. Neuropathology 28(6):577–590

11. Boer K, Crino PB, Gorter JA, Nellist M, Jansen FE, Spliet WG, van Rijen PC, Wittink FR, Breit TM, Troost D, Wadman WJ, Aronica E (2010) Gene expression analysis of tuberous sclerosis complex cortical tubers reveals increased expression of adhesion and inflammatory factors. Brain Pathol 20(4):704–719, Epub 2009 Oct 8

12. Bollo RJ, Kalhorn SP, Carlson C, Haegeli V, Devinsky O, Weiner HL (2008) Epilepsy surgery and tuberous sclerosis complex: special considerations. Neurosurg Focus 25(3):E13

13. Bombardieri R, Pinci M, Moavero R, Cerminara C, Curatolo P (2010) Early control of seizures improves long-term outcome in children with tuberous sclerosis complex. Eur J Paediatr Neurol 14(2):146–149

14. Borkowska J, Schwartz RA, Kotulska K, Jozwiak S (2011) Tuberous sclerosis complex: tumors and tumorigenesis. Int J Dermatol 50(1):13–20

15. Bourneville DM (1880) Sclérose tubéreuse des circonvolutions cérébrales. Arch Neurol 1:81–91

16. Camposano SE, Greenberg E, Kwiatkowski DJ, Thiele EA (2009) Distinct clinical characteristics of tuberous sclerosis complex patients with no mutation identified. Ann Hum Genet 73(2):141–146

17. Catania MV, D'Antoni S, Bonaccorso CM, Aronica E, Bear MF, Nicoletti F (2007) Group I metabotropic glutamate receptors: a role in neurodevelopmental disorders? Mol Neurobiol 35(3):298–307

18. Chugani DC, Chugani HT, Muzik O, Shah JR, Shah AK, Canady A, Mangner TJ, Chakraborty PK (1998) Imaging epileptogenic tubers in children with tuberous sclerosis complex using alpha-[11C]methyl-L-tryptophan positron emission tomography. Ann Neurol 44(6):858–866

19. Chu-Shore CJ, Major P, Montenegro M, Thiele E (2009) Cyst-like tubers are associated with TSC2 and epilepsy in tuberous sclerosis complex. Neurology 72(13):1165–1169

20. Chu-Shore CJ, Frosch MP, Grant PE, Thiele EA (2009) Progressive multifocal cystlike cortical tubers in tuberous sclerosis complex: clinical and neuropathologic findings. Epilepsia 50(12):2648–2651

21. Chu-Shore CJ, Major P, Camposano S, Muzykewicz D, Thiele EA (2010) The natural history of epilepsy in tuberous sclerosis complex. Epilepsia 51(7):1236–1241

22. Chu-Shore CJ, Thiele EA (2011) Tuberous sclerosis complex. In: Shorvon SD, Andermann F, Guerrini R (eds) The causes of epilepsy. Cambridge University Press, Cambridge, pp 177–182

23. Connolly MB, Hendson G, Steinbok P (2006) Tuberous sclerosis complex: a review of the management of epilepsy with emphasis on surgical aspects. Childs Nerv Syst 22(8):896–908

24. Cook T, Joshi C (2011) Gelastic seizures in tuberous sclerosis complex: case report and literature review. J Child Neurol 26(1):83–86

25. Cossu M, Cardinale F, Colombo N, Mai R, Nobili L, Sartori I, Lo Russo G (2005) Stereoelectroencephalography in the presurgical evaluation of children with drug-resistent focal epilepsy. J Neurosurg (Pediatrics 4) 103:333–343
26. Cossu M, Cardinale F, Castana L, Citterio A, Francione S, Tassi L, Benabid AL, Lo Russo G (2005) Stereoelectroencephalography in the presurgical evaluation of focal epilepsy: retrospective analysis of 215 procedures. Neurosurgery 57:706–718
27. Curatolo P, Verdecchia M, Bombardieri R (2001) Vigabatrin for tuberous sclerosis complex. Brain Dev 23(7):649–653
28. Curatolo P, Seri S, Verdecchia M, Bombardieri R (2001) Infantile spasms in tuberous sclerosis complex. Brain Dev 23(7):502–507
29. Curatolo P, Verdecchia M, Bombardieri R (2002) Tuberous sclerosis complex: a review of neurological aspects. Eur J Paediatr Neurol 6(1):15–23
30. Curatolo P, Porfirio MC, Manzi B, Seri S (2004) Autism in tuberous sclerosis. Eur J Paediatr Neurol 8:327–332
31. Curatolo P, Bombardieri R, Verdecchia M, Seri S (2005) Intractable seizures in tuberous sclerosis complex: from molecular pathogenesis to the rationale for treatment. J Child Neurol 20(4):318–325
32. Curatolo P, Bombardieri R, Jozwiak S (2008) Tuberous sclerosis. Lancet 372(9639):657–668
33. Curatolo P, Napolioni V, Moavero R (2010) Autism spectrum disorders in tuberous sclerosis: pathogenetic pathways and implications for treatment. J Child Neurol 25(7):873–880
34. Curatolo P (2010) Intractable epilepsy in tuberous sclerosis: is the tuber removal not enough? Dev Med Child Neurol 2(11):987
35. Cusmai R, Chiron C, Curatolo P, Dulac O, Tran-Dinh S (1990) Topographic comparative study of magnetic resonance imaging and electroencephalography in 34 children with tuberous sclerosis. Epilepsia 31(6):747–755
36. D'Argenzio L, Koch G, Bombardieri R, Mori F, Moavero R, Centonze D, Curatolo P (2009) Abnormal parieto-motor connectivity in tuberous sclerosis complex. Epilepsy Res 87(1): 102–105
37. De Vries P, Humphrey A, McCartney D, Prather P, Bolton P, Hunt A, TSC Behaviour Consensus Panel (2005) Consensus clinical guidelines for the assessment of cognitive and behavioural problems in tuberous sclerosis. Eur Child Adolesc Psychiatry 14(4):183–190
38. Di Michele F, Verdecchia M, Dorofeeva M, Costamagna L, Bernardi G, Curatolo P, Romeo E (2003) GABA(A) receptor active steroids are altered in epilepsy patients with tuberous sclerosis. J Neurol Neurosurg Psychiatry 74(5):667–670
39. Di Rocco C, Iannelli A, Marchese E (1995) On the treatment of subependymal giant cell astrocytomas and associated hydrocephalus in tuberous sclerosis. Pediatr Neurosurg 23(3): 115–121
40. Elliott RE, Carlson C, Kalhorn SP, Moshel YA, Weiner HL, Devinsky O, Doyle WK (2009) Refractory epilepsy in tuberous sclerosis: vagus nerve stimulation with or without subsequent resective surgery. Epilepsy Behav 16(3):454–460
41. Gallagher A, Chu-Shore CJ, Montenegro MA, Major P, Costello DJ, Lyczkowski DA, Muzykewicz D, Doherty C, Thiele EA (2009) Associations between electroencephalographic and magnetic resonance imaging findings in tuberous sclerosis complex. Epilepsy Res 87(2–3):197–202
42. Gallagher A, Grant EP, Madan N, Jarrett DY, Lyczkowski DA, Thiele EA (2010) MRI findings reveal three different types of tubers in patients with tuberous sclerosis complex. J Neurol 257(8):1373–1381
43. Gallagher A, Madan N, Stemmer-Rachamimov A, Thiele EA (2010) Progressive calcified tuber in a young male with tuberous sclerosis complex. Dev Med Child Neurol 52(11): 1062–1065
44. Ganji S, Hellman CD (1985) Tuberous sclerosis: long-term follow-up and longitudinal electroencephalographic study. Clin Electroencephalogr 16(4):219–224
45. Grajkowska W, Kotulska K, Jurkiewicz E, Matyja E (2010) Brain lesions in tuberous sclerosis complex. Review. Folia Neuropathol 48(3):139–149

46. Gupta A (2009) "Epilepsy surgery recipes galore": in quest for the epileptogenic tuber in tuberous sclerosis complex. Epileptic Disord 11(1):80–81
47. Hirose T, Scheithauer BW, Lopes MB, Gerber HA, Altermatt HJ, Hukee MJ, VandenBerg SR, Charlesworth JC (1995) Tuber and subependymal giant cell astrocytoma associated with tuberous sclerosis: an immunohistochemical, ultrastructural, and immunoelectron and microscopic study. Acta Neuropathol 90(4):387–399
48. Hofbauer GF, Marcollo-Pini A, Corsenca A, Kistler AD, French LE, Wüthrich RP, Serra AL (2008) The mTOR inhibitor rapamycin significantly improves facial angiofibroma lesions in a patient with tuberous sclerosis. Br J Dermatol 159(2):473–475
49. Hollanda FJCS, Hollanda GMP (1980) Tuberous sclerosis. Neurosurgical indications in intraventricular tumors. Neurosurg Rev 3:139–150
50. Holmes GL, Stafstrom CE; Tuberous Sclerosis Study Group (2007) Tuberous sclerosis complex and epilepsy: recent developments and future challenges. Epilepsia 48(4):617–630
51. Hou L, Klann E (2004) Activation of the phosphoinositide 3-kinase-Akt-mammalian target of rapamycin signaling pathway is required for metabotropic glutamate receptor-dependent longterm depression. J Neurosci 24(28):6352–6361
52. Humphrey A, Williams J, Pinto E, Bolton PF (2004) A prospective longitudinal study of early cognitive development in tuberous sclerosis - a clinic based study. Eur Child Adolesc Psychiatry 13(3):159–165
53. Jacobs J, Rohr A, Moeller F, Boor R, Kobayashi E, LeVan Meng P, Stephani U, Gotman J, Siniatchkin M (2008) Evaluation of epileptogenic networks in children with tuberous sclerosis complex using EEG-fMRI. Epilepsia 49(5):816–825
54. Jansen FE, van Huffelen AC, Bourez-Swart M, van Nieuwenhuizen O (2005) Consistent localization of interictal epileptiform activity on EEGs of patients with tuberous sclerosis complex. Epilepsia 46(3):415–419
55. Jansen FE, van Huffelen AC, Algra A, van Nieuwenhuizen O (2007) Epilepsy surgery in tuberous sclerosis: a systematic review. Epilepsia 48(8):1477–1484
56. Jansen FE, Braams O, Vincken KL, Algra A, Anbeek P, Jennekens-Schinkel A, Halley D, Zonnenberg BA, van den Ouweland A, van Huffelen AC, van Nieuwenhuizen O, Nellist M (2008) Overlapping neurologic and cognitive phenotypes in patients with TSC1 or TSC2 mutations. Neurology 70(12):908–915
57. Jansen FE, Vincken KL, Algra A, Anbeek P, Braams O, Nellist M, Zonnenberg BA, Jennekens-Schinkel A, van den Ouweland A, Halley D, van Huffelen AC, van Nieuwenhuizen O (2008) Cognitive impairment in tuberous sclerosis complex is a multifactorial condition. Neurology 70(12):916–923
58. Jeste SS, Sahin M, Bolton P, Ploubidis GB, Humphrey A (2008) Characterization of autism in young children with tuberous sclerosis complex. J Child Neurol 23(5):520–525
59. Joinson C, O'Callaghan FJ, Osborne JP, Martyn C, Harris T, Bolton PF (2003) Learning disability and epilepsy in an epidemiological sample of individuals with tuberous sclerosis complex. Psychol Med 33(2):335–344
60. Józwiak S, Schwartz RA, Janniger CK, Bielicka-Cymerman J (2000) Usefulness of diagnostic criteria of tuberous sclerosis complex in pediatric patients. J Child Neurol 15(10):652–659
61. Kaczorowska M, Jurkiewicz E, Doma ska-Pakieła D, Syczewska M, Lojszczyk B, Chmielewski D, Kotulska K, Kuczy ski D, Kmie T, Dunin-W sowicz D, Kasprzyk-Obara J, Jó wiak S (2011) Cerebral tuber count and its impact on mental outcome of patients with tuberous sclerosis complex. Epilepsia 52(1):22–27
62. Kagawa K, Chugani DC, Asano E, Juhász C, Muzik O, Shah A, Shah J, Sood S, Kupsky WJ, Mangner TJ, Chakraborty PK, Chugani HT (2005) Epilepsy surgery outcome in children with tuberous sclerosis complex evaluated with alpha-[11C]methyl-L-tryptophan positron emission tomography (PET). J Child Neurol 20(5):429–438
63. Karenfort M, Kruse B, Freitag H, Pannek H, Tuxhorn I (2002) Epilepsy surgery outcome in children with focal epilepsy due to tuberous sclerosis complex. Neuropediatrics 33(5): 255–261
64. Kassiri J, Snyder TJ, Bhargava R, Wheatley BM, Sinclair DB (2011) Cortical tubers, cognition, and epilepsy in tuberous sclerosis. Pediatr Neurol 44(5):328–332

65. Kaufmann R, Kornreich L, Goldberg-Stern H (2009) Unusual clinical presentation of tuberless tuberous sclerosis complex. J Child Neurol 24(3):361–364
66. Kossoff EH, Vining EP, Pillas DJ, Pyzik PL, Avellino AM, Carson BS, Freeman JM (2003) Hemispherectomy for intractable unihemispheric epilepsy etiology vs outcome. Neurology 61(7):887–890
67. Kossoff EH (2010) Infantile spasms. Neurologist 16(2):69–75
68. Lachhwani DK, Pestana E, Gupta A, Kotagal P, Bingaman W, Wyllie E (2005) Identification of candidates for epilepsy surgery in patients with tuberous sclerosis. Neurology 64(9): 1651–1654
69. Lazarowski AJ, Lubieniecki FJ, Camarero SA, Pomata HH, Bartuluchi MA, Sevlever G, Taratuto AL (2006) New proteins configure a brain drug resistance map in tuberous sclerosis. Pediatr Neurol 34(1):20–24
70. Leal AJ, Dias AI, Vieira JP, Moreira A, Távora L, Calado E (2008) Analysis of the dynamics and origin of epileptic activity in patients with tuberous sclerosis evaluated for surgery of epilepsy. Clin Neurophysiol 119(4):853–861
71. Leiphart JW, Peacock WJ, Mathern GW (2001) Lobar and multilobar resections for medically intractable pediatric epilepsy. Pediatr Neurosurg 34(6):311–318
72. Mackay MT, Becker LE, Chuang SH, Otsubo H, Chuang NA, Rutka J, Ben-Zeev B, Snead OC 3rd, Weiss SK (2003) Malformations of cortical development with balloon cells: clinical and radiologic correlates. Neurology 60(4):580–587
73. Madhavan D, Weiner HL, Carlson C, Devinsky O, Kuzniecky R (2007) Local epileptogenic networks in tuberous sclerosis complex: a case review. Epilepsy Behav 11(1):140–146
74. Madhavan D, Schaffer S, Yankovsky A, Arzimanoglou A, Renaldo F, Zaroff CM, LaJoie J, Weiner HL, Andermann E, Franz DN, Leonard J, Connolly M, Cascino GD, Devinsky O (2007) Surgical outcome in tuberous sclerosis complex: a multicenter survey. Epilepsia 48(8):1625–1628
75. Major P, Thiele EA (2008) Vagus nerve stimulation for intractable epilepsy in tuberous sclerosis complex. Epilepsy Behav 13:357–360
76. Major P, Rakowski S, Simon MV, Cheng ML, Eskandar E, Baron J, Leeman BA, Frosch MP, Thiele EA (2009) Are cortical tubers epileptogenic? Evidence from electrocorticography. Epilepsia 50(1):147–154
77. Maldonado M, Baybis M, Newman D, Kolson DL, Chen W, McKhann G 2nd, Gutmann DH, Crino PB (2003) Expression of ICAM-1, TNF-alpha, NF kappa B, and MAP kinase in tubers of the tuberous sclerosis complex. Neurobiol Dis 14(2):279–290
78. Matsuo N, Imamura A, Ito R, Sugawara K, Takahashi Y, Kondo N (2007) The correlation between 1H-MR spectroscopy and clinical manifestation with tuberous sclerosis complex. Neuropediatrics 38(3):126–129
79. Milh M, Villeneuve N, Chapon F, Pineau S, Lamoureux S, Livet MO, Bartoli C, Hugonenq C, Mancini J, Chabrol B, Girard N (2009) Transient brain magnetic resonance imaging hyperintensity in basal ganglia and brain stem of epileptic infants treated with vigabatrin. J Child Neurol 24(3):305–315
80. Mizuguchi M, Takashima S (2001) Neuropathology of tuberous sclerosis. Brain Dev 23(7):508–515
81. Moavero R, Cerminara C, Curatolo P (2010) Epilepsy secondary to tuberous sclerosis: lessons learned and current challenges. Childs Nerv Syst 26(11):1495–1504
82. Moavero R, Pinci M, Bombardieri R, Curatolo P (2011) The management of subependymal giant cell tumors in tuberous sclerosis: a clinician's perspective. Childs Nerv Syst 27:1203–1210
83. Moshel YA, Elliott R, Teutonico F, Sellin J, Carlson C, Devinsky O, Weiner HL (2010) Do tubers contain function? Resection of epileptogenic foci in perirolandic cortex in children with tuberous sclerosis complex. Epilepsia 51(7):1242–1251
84. Muncy J, Butler IJ, Koenig MK (2009) Rapamycin reduces seizure frequency in tuberous sclerosis complex. J Child Neurol 24(4):477
85. Napolioni V, Curatolo P (2008) Genetics and molecular biology of tuberous sclerosis complex. Curr Genomics 9(7):475–487

86. Napolioni V, Moavero R, Curatolo P (2009) Recent advances in neurobiology of tuberous sclerosis complex. Brain Dev 31(2):104–113
87. O'Connor SE, Kwiatkowski DJ, Roberts PS, Wollmann RL, Huttenlocher PR (2003) A family with seizures and minor features of tuberous sclerosis and a novel TSC2 mutation. Neurology 61(3):409–412
88. Ohta Y, Nariai T, Akimoto H, Shimohira M, Sugimoto J, Ohno K, Senda M, Hirakawa K (2001) Tuberous sclerosis: epileptogenicity and multimodal presurgical evaluations. Childs Nerv Syst 17(6):313–319
89. Osborne JP, Merrifield J, O'Callaghan FJK (2008) Tuberous sclerosis – what's new? Arch Dis Child 93(9):728–731
90. Park SH, Pepkowitz SH, Kerfoot C, De Rosa MJ, Poukens V, Wienecke R, DeClue JE, Vinters HV (1997) Tuberous sclerosis in a 20-week gestation fetus: immunohistochemical study. Acta Neuropathol 94(2):180–186
91. Parain D, Penniello MJ, Berquen P, Delangre T, Billard C, Murphy JV (2001) Vagal nerve stimulation in tuberous sclerosis complex patients. Pediatr Neurol 25:213–216
92. Pascual-Castroviejo I (2008) Vascular birth marks of infancy: PHACE association (Pascual-Castroviejo type II syndrome and Cobb syndrome). In: Ruggieri M, Pascual-Castroviejo I, Di Rocco C (eds) Neurocutaneous disorders: phakomatosis and hamartoneoplastic syndromes. Springer, Wien/New York, pp 19–49
93. Pascual-Castroviejo I, Alvarez-Linera J, Coya J, Viaño J, Pascual-Pascual SI, Velázquez-Fragua R, López-Gutiérrez JC (2011) Pascual-Castroviejo type II syndrome (P-CIIS). Importance of the presence of persistent embryonic arteries. Childs Nerv Syst 27(4):617–625
94. Pascual-Castroviejo I (2011) Neurosurgical treatment of tuberous sclerosis complex lesions. Childs Nerv Syst 27(8):1211–1219
95. Pellizzi GB (1901) Contributo allo studio dell'idiozia. Riv Sper Freniat 27:265–269
96. Prather P, de Vries PJ (2004) Behavioral and cognitive aspects of tuberous sclerosis complex. J Child Neurol 19(9):666–674
97. Roach ES, DiMario FJ, Kandt RS, Northrup H (1999) Tuberous sclerosis consensus conference: recommendations for diagnostic evaluation. National Tuberous Sclerosis Association. J Child Neurol 14(6):401–407
98. Romanelli P, Najjar S, Weiner HL, Devinsky O (2002) Epilepsy surgery in tuberous sclerosis: multistage procedures with bilateral or multilobar foci. J Child Neurol 17(9):689–692
99. Romanelli P, Verdecchia M, Rodas R, Seri S, Curatolo P (2004) Epilepsy surgery for tuberous sclerosis. Pediatr Neurol 31(4):239–247
100. Roth J, Olasunkanmi A, Macallister WS, Weil E, Uy CC, Devinsky O, Weiner HL (2011) Quality of life following epilepsy surgery for children with tuberous sclerosis complex. Epilepsy Behav 20(3):561–565
101. Ruggieri M, Hupadhyaya M, Di Rocco C, Gabriele A, Pascual-Castroviejo I (2008) Neurofibromatosis type I and related disorders. In: Ruggieri M, Pascual-Castroviejo I, Di Rocco C (eds) Neurocutaneous disorders: phakomatosis and hamartoneoplastic syndromes. Springer, Wien/New York, pp 51–151
102. Schwartz RA, Fernández G, Kotulska K, Jó wiak S (2007) Tuberous sclerosis complex: advances in diagnosis, genetics, and management. J Am Acad Dermatol 57(2):189–202
103. Sosunov AA, Wu X, Weiner HL, Mikell CB, Goodman RR, Crino PD, McKhann GM 2nd (2008) Tuberous sclerosis: a primary pathology of astrocytes? Epilepsia 49(Suppl 2):53–62
104. Staley BA, Vail EA, Thiele EA (2011) Tuberous sclerosis complex: diagnostic challenges, presenting symptoms, and commonly missed signs. Pediatrics 127(1):e117–e125
105. Sugiyama I, Imai K, Yamaguchi Y, Ochi A, Akizuki Y, Go C, Akiyama T, Snead OC 3rd, Rutka JT, Drake JM, Widjaja E, Chuang SH, Cheyne D, Otsubo H (2009) Localization of epileptic foci in children with intractable epilepsy secondary to multiple cortical tubers by using synthetic aperture magnetometry kurtosis. J Neurosurg Pediatr 4(6):515–522
106. Talos DM, Kwiatkowski DJ, Cordero K, Black PM, Jensen FE (2008) Cell-specific alterations of glutamate receptor expression in tuberous sclerosis complex cortical tubers. Ann Neurol 63(4):454–465

107. Tavazoie SF, Alvarez VA, Ridenour DA, Kwiatkowski DJ, Sabatini BL (2005) Regulation of neuronal morphology and function by the tumor suppressors Tsc1 and Tsc2. Nat Neurosci 8(12):1727–1734
108. Teutonico F, Mai R, Devinsky O, Lo Russo G, Weiner HL, Borrelli P, Balottin U, Veggiotti P (2008) Epilepsy surgery in tuberous sclerosis complex: early predictive elements and outcome. Childs Nerv Syst 24(12):1437–1445
109. Thapa M, Khanna PC (2010) Vigabatrin-associated diffusion MRI abnormalities in tuberous sclerosis. Pediatr Radiol 40(Suppl 1):S153
110. Toering ST, Boer K, de Groot M, Troost D, Heimans JJ, Spliet WG, van Rijen PC, Jansen FE, Gorter JA, Reijneveld JC, Aronica E (2009) Expression patterns of synaptic vesicle protein 2A in focal cortical dysplasia and TSC-cortical tubers. Epilepsia 50(6):1409–1418
111. Valencia I, Legido A, Yelin K, Khurana D, Kothare SV, Katsetos CD (2006) Anomalous inhibitory circuits in cortical tubers of human tuberous sclerosis complex associated with refractory epilepsy: aberrant expression of parvalbumin and calbindin-D28k in dysplastic cortex. J Child Neurol 21(12):1058–1063
112. van der Heide A, van Huffelen AC, Spetgens WP, Ferrier CH, van Nieuwenhuizen O, Jansen FE (2010) Identification of the epileptogenic zone in patients with tuberous sclerosis: concordance of interictal and ictal epileptiform activity. Clin Neurophysiol 121(6):842–847
113. Vigliano P, Canavese C, Bobba B, Genitori L, Papalia F, Padovan S, Forni M (2002) Transmantle dysplasia in tuberous sclerosis: clinical features and surgical outcome in four children. J Child Neurol 17(10):752–758
114. Weiner HL (2004) Tuberous sclerosis and multiple tubers: localizing the epileptogenic zone. Epilepsia 45(4):41–42
115. Westmoreland B (1999) The electroencephalogram in tuberous sclerosis. In: Gomez MR, Sampson JR, Whittemore VH (eds) Tuberous sclerosis complex: developmental perspective in psychiatry, 3rd edn. Oxford University Press, New York, pp 63–74
116. White R, Hua Y, Scheithauer B, Lynch DR, Henske EP, Crino PB (2001) Selective alterations in glutamate and GABA receptor subunit mRNA expression in dysplastic neurons and giant cells of cortical tubers. Ann Neurol 49(1):67–78
117. Willmore LJ, Abelson MB, Ben-Menachem E, Pellock JM, Shields WD (2009) Vigabatrin: 2008 update. Epilepsia 50(2):163–173
118. Wong M, Ess KC, Uhlmann EJ, Jansen LA, Li W, Crino PB, Mennerick S, Yamada KA, Gutmann DH (2003) Impaired glial glutamate transport in a mouse tuberous sclerosis epilepsy model. Ann Neurol 54(2):251–256
119. Wu JY, Sutherling WW, Koh S, Salamon N, Jonas R, Yudovin S, Sankar R, Shields WD, Mathern GW (2006) Magnetic source imaging localizes epileptogenic zone in children with tuberous sclerosis complex. Neurology 66(8):1270–1272
120. Wu JY, Salamon N, Kirsch HE, Mantle MM, Nagarajan SS, Kurelowech L, Aung MH, Sankar R, Shields WD, Mathern GW (2010) Noninvasive testing, early surgery, and seizure freedom in tuberous sclerosis complex. Neurology 74(5):392–398
121. Yapici Z, Dörtcan N, Baykan BB, Okan F, Dinçer A, Baykal C, Eraksoy M, Roach S (2007) Neurological aspects of tuberous sclerosis in relation to MRI/MR spectroscopy findings in children with epilepsy. Neurol Res 29(5):449–454
122. Zamponi N, Petrelli C, Passamonti C, Moavero R, Curatolo P (2010) Vagus nerve stimulation for refractory epilepsy in tuberous sclerosis. Pediatr Neurol 43(1):29–34
123. Zaroff CM, Devinsky O, Miles D, Barr WB (2004) Cognitive and behavioral correlates of tuberous sclerosis complex. J Child Neurol 19(11):847–852
124. Zaroff CM, Barr WB, Carlson C, LaJoie J, Madhavan D, Miles DK, Nass R, Devinsky O (2006) Mental retardation and relation to seizure and tuber burden in tuberous sclerosis complex. Seizure 15(7):558–562
125. Zeng LH, Xu L, Gutmann DH, Wong M (2008) Rapamycin prevents epilepsy in a mouse model of tuberous sclerosis complex. Ann Neurol 63(4):444–453

Critical Review of Palliative Surgical Techniques for Intractable Epilepsy

Susanne Fauser and Josef Zentner

Contents

Abstract Approximately one third of epilepsy patients are not adequately treatable by antiepileptic medication. Curative resective epilepsy surgery can be performed in only a subgroup of these pharmacoresistent patients in whom the epileptogenic focus is localizable and does not overlap with eloquent brain areas. To the remaining patients (with bilateral or multiple epileptogenic foci, with epilepsy onset in eloquent areas, or with no identifiable epileptogenic focus) palliative epilepsy surgery can be offered if they suffer from disabling seizures. Standard palliative procedures currently comprise corpus callosotomy, multiple subpial transections, and vagus nerve stimulation. New approaches such as focus distant deep brain stimulation or direct stimulation of the hippocampus have gained the most interest. Feasibility studies, small pilot studies, and, recently, larger multicenter trials showed

S. Fauser (✉)
Department of Neurosurgery, Epilepsy Center, University of Freiburg,
Breisacher Str. 64, 79106 Freiburg, Germany
e-mail: susanne.fauser@uniklinik-freiburg.de

J. Zentner
Department of Neurosurgery, University of Freiburg,
Freiburg, Germany

N. Akalan, C. Di Rocco (eds.), *Pediatric Epilepsy Surgery*,
Advances and Technical Standards in Neurosurgery,
DOI 10.1007/978-3-7091-1360-8_7, © Springer-Verlag Wien 2012

that direct brain stimulation shall be considered a potential helpful procedure in the field of palliative surgery. Moreover, with the increasing use of stereo-EEG in invasive video-EEG monitoring, stereo-EEG-guided thermocoagulation has the potential for a promising new treatment option in patients not amenable to resective epilepsy surgery. There is no general consensus on which palliative procedure is most effective in patients with difficult-to-treat epilepsy syndromes. The decision must be based on individual factors of a given patient. This review summarizes experience with palliative approaches collected in adult and pediatric patient series over the past decades and may help to thoroughly balance beneficial effects and risks of each procedure.

Keywords Palliative epilepsy surgery • Corpus callosotomy • Vagal nerve stimulation • Multiple subpial transections • Thermocoagulation • Deep brain stimulation

Introduction

Epilepsy is one of the most common neurological diseases with a prevalence of about 1 % in the world's population. Forty-seven percent of epilepsy patients become seizure-free with the first antiepileptic medication in monotherapy, and an additional 14 % of epilepsy patients will obtain seizure freedom with a second drug in monotherapy. The remaining patients are difficult to treat and often receive polytherapy [59]. Approximately one third of patients do not respond adequately to antiepileptic drugs. Even though many new antiepileptic drugs have been developed during the last 20 years, the percentage of patients with medically intractable epilepsy has not profoundly changed.

A special subgroup of these pharmacoresistent patients with focal epilepsy is amenable to curative epilepsy surgery. However, resective epilepsy surgery cannot be performed in patients in whom no epileptic focus is identifiable or a resection of the epileptogenic focus would imply severe functional impairments (e.g., speech and memory deficits, impairment of motor functions).

Severe and uncurable epilepsy syndromes often manifest in early childhood. In these patients, multifocal or large and often not localizable epileptogenic foci predispose the patient to rapid generalization of epileptic discharges and to harmful tonic or atonic drop attacks. If disabling seizures persist despite optimal medical treatment, several palliative surgical procedures can be proposed with the aim of decreasing seizure frequency and to improve quality of life. Among these procedures, we review disconnective procedures such as corpus callosotomy and multiple subpial transections, various stimulation procedures (vagal nerve stimulation, focus distant deep brain stimulation, hippocampal stimulation, responsive direct cortical stimulation), and stereo-EEG-guided thermocoagulation. For each procedure, the techniques, indications, and outcomes are described.

Detailed Review of the Literature

References for this review were identified by searches of PubMed using the terms "callosotomy," "multiple subpial transection and epilepsy," "vagus nerve stimulation and epilepsy," "brain stimulation and epilepsy," "thermocoagulation and epilepsy," and "palliative surgery and epilepsy" from January 2000 until December 2010. Further articles were identified from the references of the selected studies.

Corpus Callosotomy

History

Corpus callosotomy is the palliative procedure with the longest tradition. It was introduced in 1940 as a palliative treatment option for intractable seizures by Van Wagenen and Herren [126]. In 1975, Wilson et al. [136] were the first to use the operating microscope and developed microsurgical techniques for partial and complete callosotomy. Since then, some details of the surgical techniques have been modified [28, 31, 74, 76]. The rationale of seizure reduction by callosotomy is based on the hypothesis that the corpus callosum is the most important pathway for interhemispheric spread of epileptic activity. A disconnection of both hemispheres by a corpus callosotomy impedes rapid bilateral synchronization of epileptic discharges.

Indications

In general, corpus callosotomy successfully treats a wide variety of seizures and epilepsy syndromes and has been accepted as a palliative surgical procedure for patients with disabling seizures who are not amenable to focal resections.

Tonic and atonic drop attacks are the most common indication for corpus callosotomy [24, 43, 55, 70, 71, 73, 118, 119]. Thus, corpus callosotomy is a treatment option in children with Lennox-Gastaut syndrome comprising tonic, atonic, or tonic-clonic seizures [24, 60, 96, 134]. Further candidates for corpus callosotomy are patients with (a) recurrent episodes of status epilepticus [70, 71], (b) partial (mainly frontal) seizure onset and rapid secondary generalization, (c) no obvious epileptogenic focus, and (d) multifocal or widespread lesions (e.g., tuberous sclerosis, hemimegalencephaly) [55, 65, 70, 99]. Moreover, few publications report a marked benefit in patients with medically refractory idiopathic epilepsy with generalized tonic-clonic and absence of seizures [23, 52].

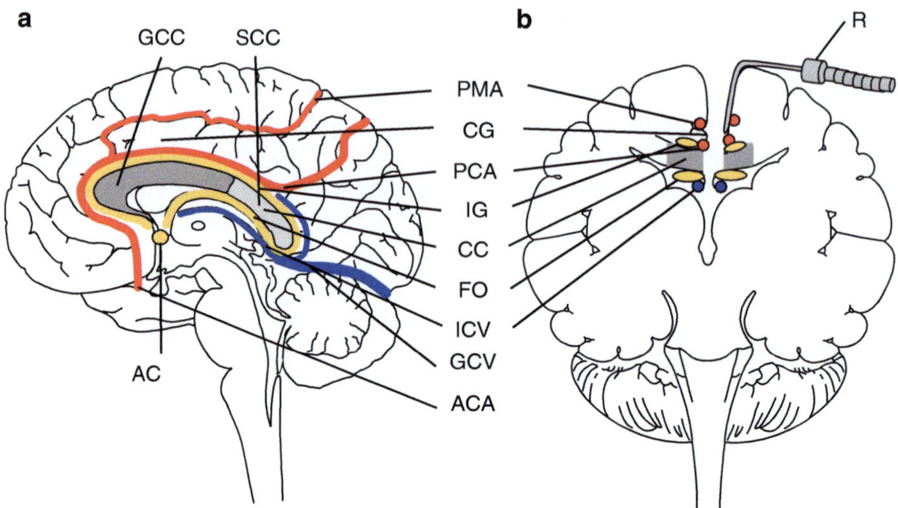

Fig. 1 Illustration of corpus callosotomy. (**a**) Sagittal view of a brain in midline. Anterior two-third callosotomy is indicated in *dark gray*, and posterior one-third callosotomy is indicated in *light gray*. (**b**) The left vertex is gently pushed aside with a self-retaining retractor (*R*). *AC* anterior commissure, *ACA* anterior cerebral artery, *CC* corpus callosum, *CG* cingulate gyrus, *FO* fornix, *GCV* great cerebral vein of Galen, *GCC* genu corporis callosi, *ICV* internal cerebral vein, *IG* indusium griseum, *PCA* pericallosal artery, *PMA* pericallosal marginal artery, *SCC* splenium corporis callosi red color: arteries, blue color: veins, yellow color: nerval structures.

Techniques

At our institution callosotomy is performed as follows: After intubation, the patient is positioned on the operating table with the head fixed in a three-point skeletal fixation. The position is supine with 30° inclination of the head for anterior and complete callosotomy and prone 20° retroflexion of the head for posterior callosotomy. At the time of scalp incision, mannitol (1 g/kg) is administered intravenously. For an anterior callosotomy, a right frontal free bone flap measuring 5 × 5 cm and which runs 1 cm dorsal and 5 cm anterior to the bregma and slightly crosses the midline is fashioned. The corresponding bone flap for a posterior callosotomy measures 6 × 5 cm, extends 1 cm posterior to the lambda and 5 cm anterior to the lambda and slightly crosses the midline. The dura is opened in a curvilinear fashion and reflected to the sagittal sinus. At this point, the operation microscope is used.

While dissecting the interhemispheric fissure, it may be necessary to divide small bridging veins. However, division of larger veins posterior to the bregma is always avoided. The dissection down to the interhemispheric fissure is continued, dividing arachnoidal adhesions that are often encountered, particularly in patients who have an incomplete falx cerebri and at the level of the cingular gyrus, until the corpus callosum is reached (Fig. 1). The corpus callosum is readily distinguished from the overlying cingulate cortex by its glistening, bright white color. The self-retaining retractor is inserted and the pericallosal arteries are identified. Further exposure of the callosum is accomplished following the pericallosal arteries anteriorly as well as posteriorly. In order to provide sufficient working space between both pericallosal arteries, small arterial vessels supplying the exposed corpus callosum as well as veins are coagulated and divided. Thereafter, the pericallosal arteries are protected with cotton wool and the retractor is adjusted over the protected artery.

Division of the corpus callosum is accomplished using a microsuction device or the cavitron ultrasonic aspirator (CUSA). The dissection is performed in the midline because on the indusium griseum, a commissural hippocampal pathway is located on both lateral surfaces of the corpus callosum. The dissection is carried down to the blue-gray lining that provides a thin barrier and which may be preserved in its integrity. In the anterior procedure, sectioning is first performed forward through the genu and rostrum until the anterior commissure, which is spared, is seen. The anterior commissure is a commissural pathway between both temporal lobes. Thereafter, sectioning of the callosal fibers is extended posteriorly as desired. When partial section is performed, a titanium clip may be placed at the posterior extent of the division to facilitate imaging of that limit and to serve as a surgical marker should a subsequent complete callosotomy be required. If complete callosotomy is intended, division is carried out through the splenium to the tentorial arachnoid until the vein of Galen is seen. While splitting the commissura fornicis, it is essential to keep the midline, thus not jeopardizing the fornix. The interhemispheric fissure is examined throughout its length to assure hemostasis. After closing the dura, the free bone flap is reimplanted, a subgaleal drain is placed, and the scalp is closed conventionally in two layers [141].

Other surgical techniques currently used may differ with respect to positioning of the patient, skin incision, extent of trephination, methods of brain relaxation, and tools used for sectioning the corpus callosum. Recently, radiosurgical callosotomy with gamma knife has been performed [16, 28, 31, 115].

Results

Outcome of Callosotomy

The postoperative outcome is highly dependent on the *seizure types* occurring in a given patient. According to recent studies of larger patient series [24, 43, 70, 118, 119], *drop attacks* best responded to corpus callosotomy: 44–84 % of patients were cured from drop attacks (tonic/atonic) and 80–99 % of patients (including those with cure from this seizure type) had at least a moderate improvement with >50 % seizure reduction. Favorable results were also obtained in patients with *secondarily generalized tonic-clonic seizures*: In 12–57 % of patients secondarily generalized seizures were completely abolished and 46–94 % of patients (including those with cure from this seizure type) showed >50 % seizure reduction. Concerning *atypical absences*, outcome was also quite satisfactory: In 20–82 % of patients, atypical absences completely stopped and 53–90 % of patients (including those with cure from this seizure type) had >50 % seizure reduction. Less impressive results were observed for *complex partial seizures*: 0–22 % of patients were free from complex partial seizures and 20–91 % of patients (including those with cure from this seizure type) had >50 % seizure relief. Also, poorer outcomes are described in *myoclonic seizures*: 0–27 % of patients were seizure free and 27–92 % of patients (including those with cure from this seizure type) had at least >50 % seizure reduction (Tables 1a and 3).

Table 1a Seizure reduction per seizure type after callosotomy

Seizure type	Seizure reduction	Maehara et al. (2001) (52 patients) (%)	Hanson et al. [43] (41 patients) (%)	Cukiert et al. [24] (76 patients) (%)	Sunaga et al. [118] (78 patients) (%)	Tanriverdi et al. [119] (95 patients) (%)
Drop attacks	Cure	80	–	–	84	44
	>50 % reduction	92	80	–	93	99
GTC	Cure	12	–	57	27	50
	>50 % reduction	61	50	57	56	94
Atypical	Cure	20	–	49	31	32
absences	>50 % reduction	53	–	82	72	90
CPS	Cure	0	–	–	14	22
	>50 % reduction	20	57	–	21	91
Myoclonic	Cure	0	–	27	–	27
seizures	>50 % reduction	27	–	73	–	92

Recent publications are listed. Consistently best results are reported in drop attacks and generalized tonic-clonic seizures

GTC generalized tonic-clonic seizures, *CPS* complex partial seizures

Table 1b Seizure reduction per seizure type after VNS in Lennox-Gastaut syndrome

Seizure type	Seizure reduction	Majoie et al. [72] (19 patients) (%)	Kostov et al. [57] (30 patients) (%)
Drop attacks	Cure	8	24
(or tonic/atonic seizures)	>50 % reduction	23	64
GTC	Cure	0	15
	>50 % reduction	10	55
Atypical absences	Cure	10	20
	>50 % reduction	40	60
CPS	Cure	20	0
	>50 % reduction	60	75
Myoclonic seizures	Cure	14	18
	>50 % reduction	57	54

Vagus nerve stimulation had a certain effect on all seizure types without any preference. More favorable results in the study by Kostov et al. may be related to a longer observation period
GTC generalized tonic-clonic seizures, *CPS* complex partial seizures

Apart from the seizure type, the *underlying pathology* may play a role in postoperative outcome. In patients with bilateral malformations of the cortical development such as diffuse cortical dysplasia, tuberous sclerosis and lissencephaly, good surgical results have been reported with callosotomy [113, 119]. In patients with temporal lobe epilepsy, however, complex partial seizures are probably not influenced by anterior callosotomy [98, 113].

The *extent of the corpus callosotomy* also influences the seizure outcome. In several outcome analyses, a complete corpus callosotomy was superior to an anterior two-thirds corpus callosotomy, but the risk of peri- and postoperative complications was also slightly higher with complete callosotomy [49, 52, 55, 100, 118, 119, 123, 138].

Further prognostic factors concerning the postoperative outcome may relate to several *EEG features*. Seizure onset with generalized slow spike-wave complexes, electrodecrement, or low-amplitude fast activity as well as *interictal* slow spike-wave activity was associated with a favorable postoperative outcome. In contrast, interictal EEG recordings revealing bilateral independent spikes have been associated with poor outcome [43].

Several studies report long-term follow-ups in patients with corpus callosotomy [50, 118, 119, 121, 123]. The observation period ranged between 1 and 25 years. All these studies agree that complete seizure freedom after corpus callosotomy is an absolute rarity and is observed in only one reported patient [123]. Considerable improvement (>50 % seizure reduction), in particular concerning the most disabling seizure types, is consistently reported in 60–76 % of patients (Table 2).

In addition to seizure reduction, several studies report improvement in overall daily functions [70, 101, 123]: Changes include improvement in hyperactivity, emotional well-being, speech functions, memory functions, attentiveness, and self-care. Younger age (<18 years) at the time of surgery was an independent predictive factor for improvement in daily functions [70, 123] but not for seizure outcome [6].

Table 2 Comparison of different palliative procedures – outcome

Approach	Percentage of seizure-free patients	Percentage of patients with >50 % seizure reduction	Comments
Callosotomy	Nearly 0	60–76	Large patient series available, considerable reduction of drop attacks and generalized tonic-clonic seizures
MST + cortical resection	42–56	80–88	Seizure relapse in 20 % of patients in a long-term outcome analysis
MST alone	0–15	45–51	Only small patient series available
VNS			Large patient series available
Retrospective studies	0–8	40–64	
Prospective studies	2	23–51	
DBS (ANT) (SANTE study)	13 (at least 6 months)	54	Only significant seizure reduction in temporal lobe CPS
SEEG-guided thermocoagulation	0	54	Only small patient series

Seizure freedom is rarely obtained by palliative procedures. Only MST in combination with cortical resection can be regarded as a curative approach. The main aim of palliative procedures is reduction of the frequency of most disabling seizures and improvement of quality of life
MST multiple subpial transections, *VNS* vagus nerve stimulation, *DBS* deep brain stimulation, *ANT* anterior nucleus of the thalamus, *SEEG* stereoelectroencephalography

Safety Aspects of Callosotomy

Most adverse effects of corpus callosotomy are temporary. Permanent neurological deficits are rare. However, the risk/benefit ratio to such therapy needs to be carefully assessed. Common adverse effects are the following:

Surgical complications: Surgical complications mainly included acute epidural hematoma, hydrocephalus, subdural cerebrospinal fluid accumulation, infections (e.g., meningitis, osteomyelitis), and deep-vein thrombosis, and occurred in 9–20 % of patients [50, 70, 71, 90, 113, 118, 119]. The mortality rate was reported at 2 % in a study from 1977 [137]. Modern techniques yielded lower rates and no deaths were reported in the recent patient series 113.

Permanent neurological deficits: Permanent neurological deficits were caused mainly by trauma, infarction, or intracerebral hemorrhage and occurred in <4 % of patients since the introduction of microsurgical techniques [71, 90].

Disconnection syndrome: Disconnection syndromes are more common with total than with anterior callosotomy. Most patients are unaware of their deficits [55]. Acute disconnection symptoms such as apathy, urinary incontinence, low verbal output, and hemineglect are very common and usually diminish by time (mean duration 16 days) [24]. Permanent disconnection syndromes are rare (3 %) and to some extent may fluctuate over years [24]. They comprise several phenomena: alien hand syndrome, dichotic listening suppression, tactile dysnomia, hemispatial neglect, nondominant hand agraphia, alexia without agraphia, and tachistoscopic visual suppression (reviewed by Jea et al. [51]). The alien hand syndrome is the most impressive disconnection syndrome, characterized by the phenomenon that the nondominant hand (or leg) acts without guidance of the patient's own will, resulting in complex involuntary movements and intermanual conflicts. Examples are involuntary unbuttoning of clothing, removing objects from tables, throwing objects or even walking in the wrong direction. In addition, apraxia and mutism have been reported.

Memory deficits: Memory deficits are rarely observed and may be related to a section of the hippocampal commissures (fornix and indusium griseum), in particular, by dissection of the splenium, due to the anatomical proximity of the fornix commissure [70, 102].

New types of seizures: The emergence of new varieties of mainly simple partial seizures has been reported [70, 123]. There may be a transient increase in focal seizures immediately after surgery, which typically resolves within 1–2 months.

Multiple Subpial Transection (MST)

History

Based on the observations that a neuronal functional unit is organized vertically [84, 85], the seizures spread horizontally [19, 133], and a minimal contiguous cortical surface area is necessary for the maintenance of cortical activity [69, 103], Morrell et al. [81] suggested a novel technique called multiple subpial transection (MST) in 1989. Vertical transections should theoretically disrupt only horizontally oriented axons and thus the spread of epileptic activity while preserving the vertically oriented architecture and cortical function.

Indications

MST has been developed for surgically intractable epilepsy with seizure foci in primary sensomotor or language areas. MST might be an effective alternative to subtotal resection of the epileptogenic zone in critical brain areas; thus, it has a role when performed in conjunction with cortical resections or lesionectomies [12, 114]. MST as stand-alone therapy, however, may be indicated only in highly selected cases. Moreover, MST has been considered effective for patients with Landau-Kleffner syndrome (LKS) [14, 39, 80].

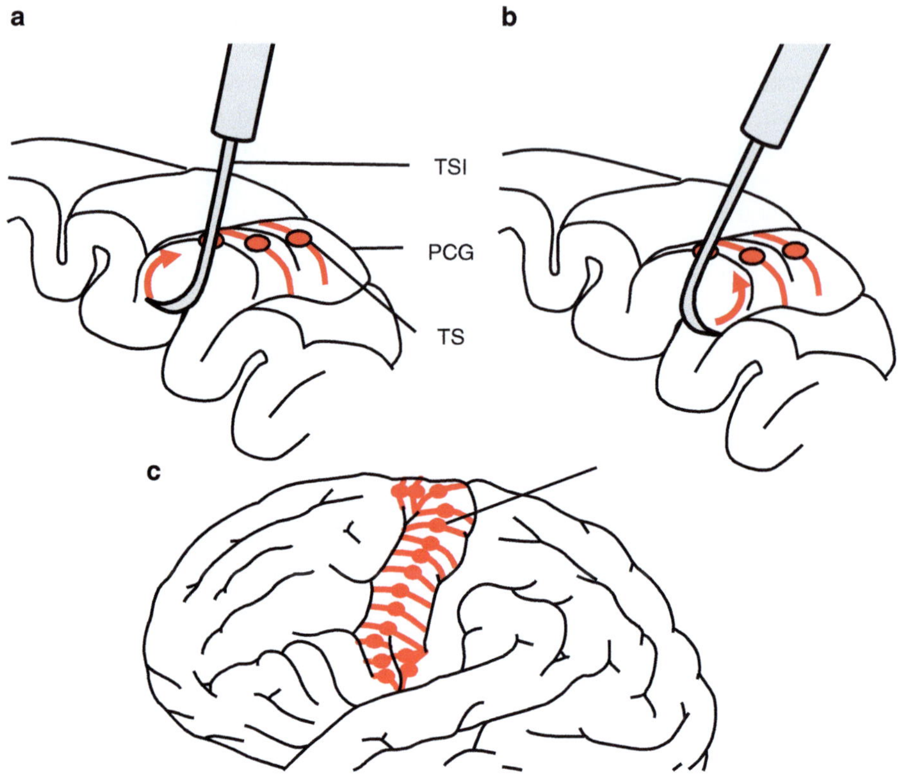

Fig. 2 Illustration of multiple subpial transections. (a) Transversal section through the cortex, demonstrating the maneuver with the transection instrument (*TSI*). The precentral gyrus (*PCG*) is entered through a point incision of the pia mater (*red point*); the instrument is gently moved along the curved tip to the opposite side of the gyrus. Thereafter, the transection (*TS, red lines*) is carried out by drawing the curved tip backward along the pia mater of the gyrus (b). The whole maneuver has to be carried out in a circle-like manner (*red arrows*). (c) The transection direction is always vertical against the surrounding sulci

Techniques

MST is conducted according to the technique of Morrell [81]. After bipolar electrocautery of points spaced approximately 5 mm apart along the edge of a given gyrus, the pia mater is sharply incised (Fig. 2). Serial MST are then performed through the incised pial points to a depth of approximately 1.5–2 cm along an axis perpendicular to the gyrus using different hooks. The tip of the knife is visualized through the pia mater as it is drawn back along the subpial space, completing the transection. Care should be taken to avoid disrupting the pia mater or catching sulcal vessels during the transection procedure. In cases wherein MST are performed in multiple contiguous gyri in one or more lobes of the brain, intraoperative ultrasonography can be used at the end of the procedure to ensure that no underlying intracerebral hematoma was created. Electrocorticography is performed before and after MST to evaluate the interictal activity and response to surgery.

Results

Outcome of MST

Effects of MST on epilepsy are reported in several patient series with variable success. In general, MST performed in combination with resections showed more favorable outcomes than MST alone. According to more recent studies and reviews [8, 12, 47, 91, 97], 42–56 % of patients became seizure-free and in 80–88 % (including seizure-free patients), seizure frequency was considerably reduced (>50 %) when MST was performed in conjunction with cortical resection. However, in the long run (observation periods of 28–89 months after surgery), 19 % of patients sustained an increase in seizure frequency several years after initial postoperative improvement [91] (Table 2).

When MST was conducted as stand-alone therapy, results were less impressive [47, 97, 111]: 0–15 % of patients became seizure-free and 45–51 % (including seizure-free patients) had >50 % seizure reduction. Only one publication [117] reported satisfactory seizure outcomes in selected patients who underwent MST without resection (Table 2).

Multiple subpial transections have been performed in small patient series with Landau-Kleffner syndrome (LKS) (Table 3). Morrell, who first described the procedure, reviewed the experience with 14 patients with LKS who underwent MST. Seventy-nine percent of the patients showed marked improvement in speech and understanding [80]. Similar successful outcomes were reported by Buelow et al. [14] and Grote et al. [39] (1999). Irwin et al. [48] reported on five children with LKS who underwent MST. Language skills improved in all children but none improved to an age-appropriate level. Seizures and behavioral disturbances were immediately ameliorated after the intervention. Cross and Neville [22], reporting on a series of ten patients, found seizure improvement in 50 % of them, 70 % showed language improvement, and some of them had significant behavioral improvement.

Safety Aspects of MST

Transient neurological deficits following MST are frequently observed and are caused by an edema. Transient hemiparesis was seen in around 60 % of patients who underwent MST of the primary motor area and mild to moderate dysphasia in approximately 60 % of patients following MST of the language area [12]. These deficits may persist from 6 weeks to 6 months [12]. Permanent neurological deficits were not or only exceptionally observed in the published patient series [86, 106, 108].

Table 3 Summary of possible indications for palliative procedures in different seizure types and syndromes

	Drop attacks (tonic/atonic)	Myoclonic seizures	Complex partial seizures	Atypical absences	Primarily generalized tonic-clonic seizures	Secondarily generalized tonic-clonic seizures	Malformations of cortical development	Seizures originating from eloquent areas	LGS	LKS
Callosotomy	+++	+	+	++	+	++	+	–	++	–
MST+cortical resection	–	–	–	–	–	–	–	+++	–	–
MST alone								+		+
VNS	+	++	++	+	+	+	(+)	+	+	?
DBS (anterior nucleus of the thalamus)	?	?	+	?	?	?	?	?	?	?

+++, >50 % seizure reduction in >75 % of patients consistently reported in all studies; ++, >50 % seizure reduction in >50 % of patients consistently reported in all studies; +, >50 % seizure reduction in >50 % of patients reported in at least one study; (+) poor or less robust results compared to other indications, ? effect not known yet

MST multiple subpial transections, *VNS* vagus nerve stimulation, *DBS* deep brain stimulation

Vagus Nerve Stimulation (VNS)

History

The idea of stimulating the vagus nerve to modify central brain activity has been pursued for over 100 years. In 1952, desynchronizing effects of vagal nerve stimulation (VNS) were noted on feline sleep spindles as well as on a strychnine model of epileptiform activity [140]. In 1988, the first stimulator was implanted in a human [95]. VNS therapy received European Community approval in 1994 and US Food and Drug Administration (FDA) approval in 1997. Meanwhile, >50,000 patients have been treated worldwide for epilepsy by VNS therapy. The exact mechanism by which VNS modulates seizures is not known. The vagus nerve projects primarily to the nucleus of the solitary tract, which has projections to multiple areas in the forebrain and brainstem, including areas involved in epileptogenesis such as thalamus, hippocampus, amygdala, and neocortex [107, 132]. It has been postulated that the anticonvulsant effect of VNS may be caused by the release of norepinephrine or its influence on the reticular activating system [58, 77].

Indications

VNS is indicated as an adjunctive therapy for reducing the frequency of seizures in adults and adolescents over 12 years of age with partial onset seizures that are refractory to antiepileptic drugs. Meanwhile, many children under 12 years of age with severe epilepsy have been treated off-label [2, 9–11, 25, 26, 27, 29, 36, 37, 42, 45, 57, 88, 112, 124, 131].

Techniques

The patient is positioned supine on the operating table with the head neutral and slightly to moderately extended. The incision is made in a skin crease or fold whenever possible (Fig. 3a). Upon completion of the cervical incision and vagus nerve isolation, either a subcutaneous or a subpectoral approach can be performed. In the subcutaneous approach, the skin incision is made in the left axilla line. A subcutaneous pocket is created directly over the pectoral muscle. In the subpectoral approach [7], the skin incision is made on the lateral border of the pectoralis major, approximately 20 cm below the level of the clavicle along a natural skin crease. The subcutaneous fat layer is then divided with monopolar cautery and with blunt dissection until the lateral border of the pectoralis is visualized. The pectoralis fascia is bluntly divided to the subpectoral fascia, and a pocket is bluntly dissected between the superior and inferior pectoralis fascia. After preparing the pocket, the generator is placed within the pocket to verify the appropriate size of the pocket and resulting skin contour and approximation at the incision. A subcutaneous tunnel is then created from

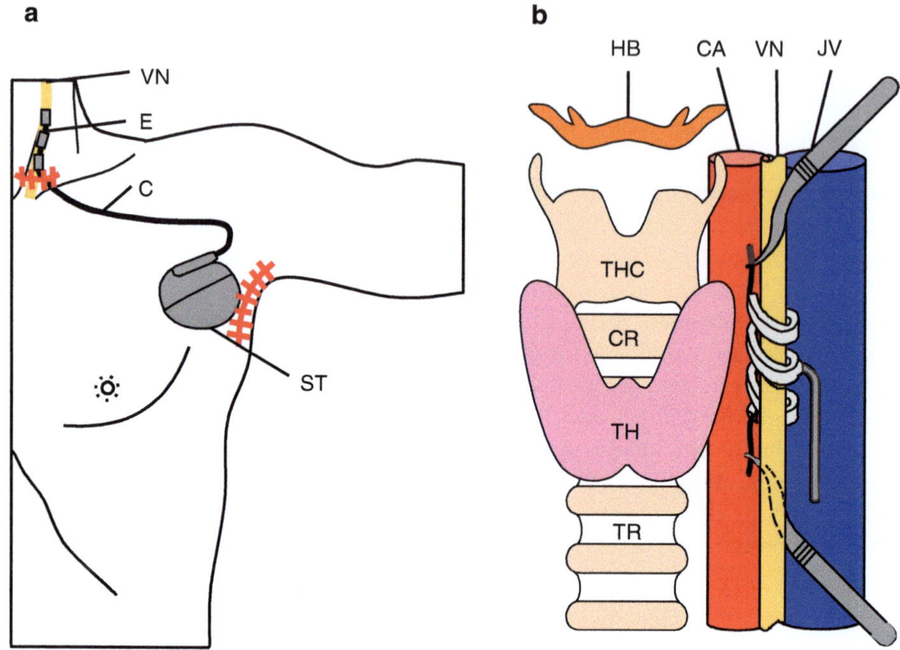

Fig. 3 Illustration of a vagus nerve stimulator implantation. (**a**) Overview of the location of the electrode contacts (*E*) at the vagus nerve (*VN*). The electrodes are connected by a subcutaneous, tunneled cable (*C*) with the stimulator unit (*ST*), which is implanted either subcutaneously or below the pectoral muscle. The *red lines* indicate skin incisions. (**b**) Illustration of the electrode placement along the vagus nerve (*VN*), which is located within a common soft tissue sheet between the carotid artery (*CA*) and jugular vein (*JV*). *CR* cricoid cartilage, *HB* hyoid bone, *TR* trachea, *TH* thyroid gland, *THC* thyroid cartilage

the chest incision to the cervical incision, and the electrode is passed and appropriately positioned around the vagus nerve (Fig. 3b). The cervical skin incision is performed in paramedian between the midline and the border of the sternocleidomastoid muscle below the height of the thyroid cartilage, preferably in a preexisting skin fold. The platysma muscle is prepared and vertically incised. Then the gap between the infrahyal and sternocleidomastoid muscle is bluntly dissected. The common soft tissue sheet of the vagus nerve, carotid artery, and jugular vein is located and incised. The vagus nerve is usually between and behind both vessels. The nerve has to be prepared, with no soft tissue left on the perineurium. Only then can the electrodes be wrapped around the nerve, as shown in Fig. 3b. The electrode wire lead is then secured to the fascia or muscle of the cervical region at two locations and attached to the generator and secured with the set screw. The generator is then placed into the chest pocket and the coil of the remaining lead is placed outside and adjacent to the body of the generator to provide extra length and protection. Thereafter, the generator is tested again to verify that the system's electrical integrity is optimal and that the impedance is within the range for appropriate stimulation function. Finally, the subpectoral or cutaneous pocket and the skin are closed with sutures.

Results

Outcome of VNS

VNS has been proven effective in medically intractable epilepsy. According to many retrospective studies reported between 1999 and 2011 [2, 8–10, 25, 29, 36, 45, 88, 110, 112, 124], 40–64 % of patients have >50 % seizure reduction and 0–8 % of patients became seizure-free. Similar positive results were reported in several registries [3, 61, 104]. Few prospective observational studies and randomized controlled trials [4, 11, 26, 27, 37, 42, 131] have demonstrated >50 % seizure reduction in 23–51 % of patients. According to these studies, approximately 2 % of patients became completely seizure-free (Table 2).

VNS has been reported to be effective in children with Lennox-Gastaut syndrome [36, 45, 57, 72, 105, 112]. In this special patient group, the responder rate (>50 % seizure reduction) was reported in 25–78 % of patients. The high variability may be a result of different group sizes (between 7 and 30 patients per group) and different observation periods. Two studies comprising larger patient numbers report also seizure reduction per seizure type [57, 72]. VNS had a certain effect on all seizure types without any preference to more disabling seizure types. Concerning (tonic and atonic) *drop attacks*, seizure freedom could be achieved in 8–24 % of patients and >50 % seizure reduction was seen in 23–64 % of patients. *Generalized tonic-clonic seizures* were completely abolished in 0–15 % and >50 % seizure reduction was achieved in 10–55 % of patients. *Atypical absences* completely ceased in 10–20 % of patients and >50 % seizure reduction was observed in 40–60 % of patients. *Complex partial seizures* were completely abolished in 0–20 % of patients and >50 % seizure reduction was seen in 60–75 % of patients. *Myoclonic seizures* were completely absent in 14–18 % of patients and >50 % seizure reduction was reported in 54–57 % of patients. The poorer results in the study by Majoie et al. [72] may be related to a relatively short observation period of 6 months (Tables 1b and 3).

Few predictors of VNS efficacy have been consistently reported in the literature. One of the most common and consistent findings is improved seizure control with increasing duration of VNS therapy [3, 27, 38, 45, 61, 87, 94]. Others have reported the following variables as predictors of improved response to VNS: focal epilepsy (eloquent) or temporal lobe epilepsy [29]; fewer failed antiepileptic drugs (AED) [104] higher baseline seizure frequency [62], prior corpus callosotomy [45, 61], higher cognitive function at baseline [1], and focal rather than generalized seizures [61]. Contradictory results were reported as to patient age at implantation [2, 25, 61] and duration of epilepsy [104, 61]. Neuronal migration disorders predicted less robust response to therapy [29].

No negative cognitive side effects have been reported with VNS. Cognition may even improve if concomitant medications can be reduced. VNS therapy promotes alertness [75], improves mood [44], and can provide quality-of-life benefits [30]. VNS may stop or shorten seizures and clusters of seizures and also may improve the postictal period [120].

Safety Aspects of VNS

The placement of a VNS device is a low-risk procedure. Infection may occur at the incision site [116]; the rate of infections is reported between 0 and 8 % (Elliott et al. 2010). There may be paralysis of the vocal cord (usually transient). Significant or permanent injury to the vagus nerve was rare (<4 %) (Elliott et al. 2010). Rarely asystole may occur in the operating room (0.1 %) [109]. Lead fracture or dislodgement from the device and battery failure can occur unrelated to the surgical procedure [45, 116].

In the long run, patients may commonly complain of voice alteration and hoarseness (19–29 %), local paresthesias, throat or neck pain (12 %), and cough (6 %). Dyspnea may be seen (3 %), as well as headaches [18, 42, 56, 83, 87, 116].

Direct and Deep Brain Stimulation for the Treatment of Epilepsy

History

For decades, the effects of electrical stimulation on brain activity have been studied. Direct stimulation of the cerebellum was reported to be effective in treating epilepsy in noncontrolled studies [21], but subsequent controlled studies in a total of 17 patients failed to show significant effects [125, 139]. Early investigations of the thalamus in animal models of epilepsy demonstrated the potential for disruption of seizures induced by both pharmacological and electrical stimulation [78, 79]. Thus, focus distant brain stimulation is supposed to modulate and/or disrupt epileptic activity in larger networks (e.g., in the circuit of Papez). Direct stimulation of the epileptogenic focus may abort epileptic discharges or chronically increase the threshold for epileptic activity.

Indications

Direct brain stimulation may be a treatment option for patients with bilateral or multiple seizure foci as well as for patients with seizure foci in eloquent brain areas. As with any new therapy, identification of ideal candidates remains challenging.

Thalamic stimulation for the treatment of epilepsy has been performed in the centromedian nucleus (Fig. 4a, [33, 127, 130]) and the anterior nucleus of the thalamus (Fig. 4b, [5, 32, 46, 54, 66, 92]).

First data from a multicenter, double-blind, randomized trial [32] showed that bilateral stimulation of the anterior nuclei of the thalamus (SANTE, Fig. 4b) is most effective in patients with temporal lobe epilepsy as opposed to extratemporal, neocortical epilepsy. Statistically significant improvement was noted in complex partial seizures (Table 3).

Deep brain stimulation (DBS) of the substantia nigra pars reticulata and the subthalamic nucleus may be an effective treatment option for patients with progressive myoclonic epilepsy in adulthood as shown in a small patient group [135].

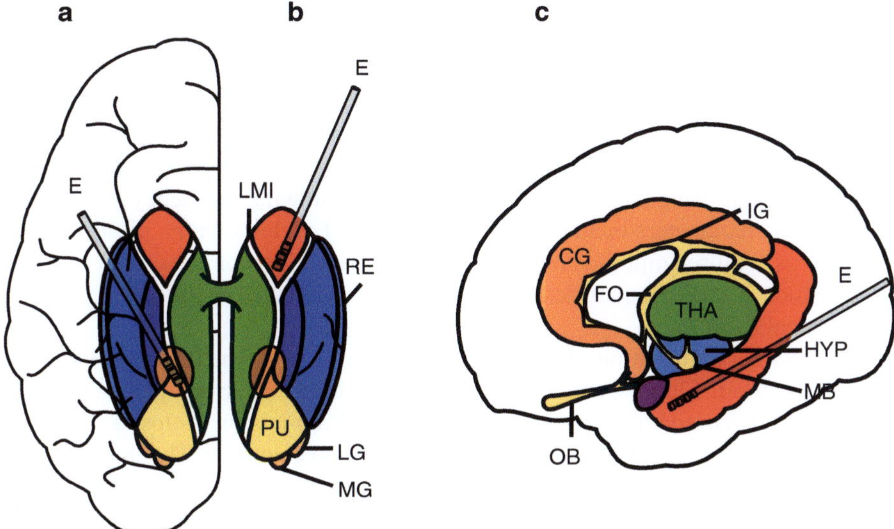

Fig. 4 Illustration of deep brain stimulation. (**a**) Overview of the locations of electrode (*E*) targets in thalamic stimulation in the centromedian nucleus (*CE*) or in the (**b**) anterior thalamic nucleus (*AN*). For anatomical orientation, other marked thalamic structures are the medial- (*ME*), ventral- (*VE*), lateral- (*LA*), pulvinar- (*PU*), lateral geniculate- (*LG*), medial geniculate (*MG*) nucleus and lamina medullaris interna (*LMI*). (**c**) Electrode (*E*) placement in hippocampal (*H*) stimulation. *A* amygdala, *CG* cingulate gyrus, *FO* fornix, *HYP* hypothalamus, *IG* indusium griseum, *MB* mammillary body, *OB* olfactory bulb, *THA* thalamus

Techniques

The procedure for electrode implantation begins with placement of the stereotactic frame under general anesthesia. After placement of an MRI localizer grid, fast spin echo inversion recovery and standard T2 high-resolution, 1-mm slice images are obtained for targeting. Computed tomography may also be a reasonable alternative for stereotactic localization. Indirect localization of the desired target can be obtained with reference to a standard stereotactic atlas by identifying the anterior and posterior commissures on axial images. Frame position relative to the AC-PC line is calculated. Direct radiographic identification of the target is also possible for most potential DBS targets, including the anterior thalamic nucleus, the subthalamic nucleus, the caudate, and the hippocampus.

The patient is fixed in a Mayfield head frame in a supine or a semisitting position. Head position is altered to optimize access to the chosen entry point. A burr hole is placed and the dura and pia are sharply incised and cauterized with care to avoid surface vessels. A guide cannula is inserted under neuronavigation from an MRI dataset. The cannula position is confirmed with fluoroscopy. A monopolar single-unit recording electrode can be introduced and used for confirmation of the targeted thalamic nucleus by recording the specific firing pattern. For targeting the anterior thalamic nucleus (AN), the lateral ventricle is invariably traversed and no unit recordings are made here. Recordings are first heard in the superficial surface of the AN. For the AN, the electrode is advanced further until recordings cease as the electrode enters the intralaminar region (Fig. 4b, LMI), in which the characteristic firing pattern ceases because the white matter generates no signal. Recordings with a different firing pattern resume as the electrode enters the dorsomedial nucleus of the thalamus (Fig. 4b, ME). For AN specifically, an additional step is used to confirm lead placement using characteristic EEG activity following frequency stimulation. Stimulation parameters include a frequency of 5–10 cycles/s with a pulse width of 90–330 µs, a pulse amplitude of 4–5 V, and total pulse duration between 3 and 10 s. Stimulation at these frequencies in the AN is associated with recruiting rhythms on the cortical EEG.

Following confirmation of EEG activity and removal of the lead, the final DBS lead is inserted. Fluoroscopy is again used to confirm electrode placement. The electrode is secured with a burr hole cap and the skin incision is closed. The same sequence of steps is used for placing the contralateral electrode. The internal pulse generator is placed the same day or 1 day later. The scalp incisions are opened and the electrode wires are identified and connected to an extension wire. These are tunneled subcutaneously to an infraclavicular position, as described in the VNS section above (Fig. 3a). Postoperatively, lead placement is confirmed with MRI or CT [63].

Results

Outcome of Direct Brain Stimulation

1. *Focus distant brain stimulation*:
   Cerebellar stimulation: A double-blind, randomized controlled pilot study of bilateral stimulation of the superomedial cerebellar cortex in five patients with medically refractory motor seizures found a significant reduction of tonic-clonic and tonic seizures over 6 months. Generalized tonic-clonic seizures were reduced after 1–2 months and continued to decrease over the first 6 months. The effect was stable over the study period of 2 years and beyond [129].

   Thalamic stimulation: Thalamic stimulation for treatment of epilepsy has been performed in the centromedian nucleus [33, 127, 130] and the anterior nucleus of the thalamus [5, 32, 46, 54, 66, 92].

   Stimulation of the *centromedian nucleus of the thalamus* has shown limited effect in humans with epilepsy: Chronic, bilateral 60-Hz stimulation of the centromedian nucleus of the thalamus in 13 patients reduced primary and secondary generalized tonic-clonic seizures but had no effect on complex partial seizures [130]. A pilot, uncontrolled nonblinded trial using continuous stimulation of the centromedian nucleus in seven patients reported significant improvement in only one patient [33].

   The *anterior nucleus of the thalamus* is an attractive target because of its close connections to the mesial temporal structures via the fornix, mammillothalamic tracts, and thalamocortical radiations. Several uncontrolled trials yielded varying results: In a publication by Andrade et al. [5], five of six patients had >50 % seizure reduction. A microthalamotomy effect on seizure expression by implantation of the electrodes alone without stimulation was suggested. In another pilot study, all four investigated patients showed >50 % seizure reduction. Lim et al. [66] investigated four patients and only one of them had a seizure reduction >50 %.

A large multicenter, double-blind, randomized trial using bilateral stimulation of the anterior nuclei of thalamus (SANTE) confirmed effectiveness (Tables 2 and 3). By 2 years, there was a 56 % median reduction in seizure frequency; 54 % of patients had a seizure reduction of >50 %, and 13 % of patients were seizure-free for at least 6 months. Patients with seizures arising from the temporal lobe(s) ($n = 66$) had a significant reduction in seizure frequency compared to baseline, whereas those with frontal ($n = 30$), parietal ($n = 5$), or occipital ($n = 4$) onsets did not demonstrate significant reduction.

Nucleus subthalamicus: The stimulation of the *subthalamic nucleus* acts via modulation of the "dorsal midbrain anticonvulsant zone." Small open-label trials have reported seizure reduction in some patients treated with this technique [17, 67]. The effect, however, seemed not to be strong enough in order to continue stimulation of the subthalamic nucleus in larger clinical studies under the stimulation parameters applied so far.

Interestingly, deep brain stimulation of the substantia nigra pars reticulata and the subthalamic nucleus may be an effective treatment option for patients with progressive myoclonic epilepsy in adulthood [135]. In all five patients in that study, significant reduction of myoclonic seizures was observed ranging between 30 and 100 %.

2. *Direct stimulation of the epileptogenic focus*:
Hippocampal stimulation: Treating temporal lobe epilepsy with stimulation seems to be attractive as it could potentially avoid memory deficits associated with surgery. Moreover, both hippocampi can be stimulated (Fig. 4c).

Uncontrolled studies with good responder rates in patients receiving continuous stimulation have been conducted as proof of principle [13, 122, 128]. Favorable results were demonstrated by Velasco et al. [128] (all nine patients were responders with >50 % seizure reduction) and by Boon et al. [13] (seven of ten patients were responders with >50 % seizure reduction). However, in the study by Tellez-Zenteno et al. [122], only one of five patients experienced >50 % seizure reduction.

Currently, larger systematic controlled studies of scheduled stimulation of the mesial temporal structures are under way (CoRaStir = prospective randomized controlled study of neurostimulation in the medial temporal lobe for patients with medial temporal lobe epilepsy; MET-TLE = randomized controlled trial of hippocampal stimulation for temporal lobe epilepsy).

Responsive cortical stimulation: Responsive neurostimulation is based on the concept that brief bursts inhibit after-discharges [20, 53, 64]. The ideal treatment scenario of responsive stimulation includes detection of an electrographic seizure by depth or cortical strip electrodes in the seizure zone before the onset of clinical symptoms. An electrical stimulus (short pulse of high-frequency stimulation) aborts the electrographic seizure and, therefore, prevents clinical symptoms. The feasibility of such devices has been demonstrated in 65 patients in whom electrodes were implanted [82]. Another feasibility study performed by a single center described a 45 % decrease in seizures in seven of eight patients with a mean follow-up of 9 months [35]. A larger pivotal double-blind controlled trial for responsive neurostimulation was performed in 109 patients; results are pending.

Responsive neurostimulation is challenging for mainly two reasons: (1) Patient-specific algorithms must be defined in order to detect early epileptiform activity in a given patient. (2) In case of incomplete stimulation of the seizure onset zone, epileptic activity may propagate from not preserve areas and expand over the whole brain.

Safety aspects of direct brain stimulation: Most common adverse effects in stimulation of the *anterior nuclei of the thalamus* are as follows:

(a) *Device-related adverse events*:
Paresthesias (18.2 %), pain at implantation site (10.9 %), and infections (12.7 %) were most commonly seen. Asymptomatic hemorrhages were noted in 4.5 % patients. Both depression and memory complaints were significantly higher in the stimulation group compared to the control group [32]. Kerrigan et al. [54] reported a 5 % risk of infection and a 5–7.5 % risk of intracerebral hemorrhage leading to clinical symptoms.

(b) *Epilepsy-related complications*:
Six percent of patients experienced new seizure types and 9 % of patients had an increase in seizure frequency compared to baseline. In 5 % of patients status epilepticus occurred: in two patients following implantation, in one patient following the initiation of stimulation after the blinded phase, and in one patient following discontinuation of stimulation. One percent of patients experienced simple partial seizures corresponding to the stimulation cycle following initiation of stimulation [32].

Most common adverse effects of *responsive neurostimulation studies* included device-related events reported in 9 % of patients, such as infections, skin erosion, cranial reconstruction, and increased seizures, all of which resolved [82]. In another responsive neurostimulation feasibility study, no serious device-related adverse event was observed [35].

One safety concern that still remains is that chronic subthreshold stimulation may induce neural injury. Experience with deep brain stimulation for patients with Parkinson's disease, however, suggests that chronic stimulation can be delivered safely [41].

SEEG-Guided Thermocoagulation

History

Developed in the 1960s for the treatment of behavioral disorders [89], stereotactic radiofrequency thermocoagulation (RFTC) lesioning was proposed for treatment of drug-resistant temporal lobe epilepsy by producing lesions in the amygdala-hippocampus structures [34]. The outcome of stereotactic RFTC targeted on a selected structure such as the amygdala or hippocampus proved definitively less favorable than that of standard surgery [93]. In recent years, the efficacy of this method has been improved by aiming at a tailored (total or partial) destruction of the epileptogenic zone using SEEG guidance [40].

Indications

Thermocoagulation may be a treatment option for patients in whom stereoelectro-encephalography (SEEG) is used for invasive video-EEG monitoring and who are not eligible for surgery because of multiple epileptogenic foci or because of the vicinity of the epileptogenic focus with respect to eloquent areas.

Techniques

The procedure is performed without anesthesia. Lesions are made using a radiofrequency lesion generator system (Radionics Medical Products, Burlington, MA) connected to the SEEG electrodes (Dixi Medical, Besancon, France). The lesions are produced between two contiguous contacts of the selected electrodes. Temperature cannot be monitored in vivo at the electrode contacts, so the lesions are made using a 50-V, 120-mA current, which was found in vitro to increase the local temperature to 78–82 °C within a few seconds. A depth EEG recording is performed for at least 5 min before and after the RFTC procedure between the two contacts used for RFTC as well as at all contacts located on the same electrode. The choice of targets depends on data from video-SEEG recordings. Criteria are low-amplitude fast-activity pattern or spike-wave discharges at onset of seizures and no clinical response to stimulation (noneloquent areas) [15].

Results

Outcome of Thermocoagulation

SEEG-guided RFTC showed a favorable benefit/risk ratio in a case series of 13 patients in whom surgery was risky or not feasible. Seven of these patients (54 %) benefited from RFTC, with a reduction of >50 % in seizure frequency [15]. Best results were obtained in patients with malformations of the cortical development (dysplasia and heterotopia) [68, 15] (Table 2).

Conversely, results of RFTC in patients eligible for lesionectomy are clearly inferior to those of surgery. Thus, SEEG-guided RFTC is not recommended as an alternative to resective surgery.

Safety Aspects of Thermocoagulation

In the above-mentioned case series, complications were rare. No permanent neuro-logical or cognitive impairment occurred after any procedure. Three of 43 patients showed transient adverse effects. Dysesthesia of the mouth occurred following intrainsular RFTC in two patients, and motor apraxia in the left hand occurred fol-lowing RFTC in the right supplementary motor area in one patient [15].

Summary, Conclusions and Proposals for the Future

Several surgical options exist for patients with medically intractable epilepsy in whom the epileptogenic focus cannot be surgically removed and in whom very dis-abling seizures persist despite optimal pharmacotherapy. These techniques allow a reduction of seizure frequency but do not cure the patient. The first-line aim is to ameliorate quality of life. The choice of the individually adequate palliative proce-dure depends on several factors. A thorough risk/benefit assessment is necessary and several points should be taken into consideration.

First, evidence base and experience concerning outcomes and long-term effects vary remarkably among the different palliative approaches. Corpus callosotomy and VNS have been performed in large patient series and long-term follow-up analyses are available. For VNS, randomized and double-blinded trials exist. Deep brain stimulation, on the other hand, is an emerging treatment option for medically intrac-table epilepsy. The best targets and modes of stimulation are still under investiga-tion. Larger, more well-controlled studies are necessary.

Second, the most disabling seizure types, epilepsy syndromes, or other patient-specific characteristics should be considered when deciding on the best palliative surgical technique. Tables 1a, b, 2, and 3 summarize different seizure types and epilepsy syndromes and the respective responsiveness to different palliative surgical techniques reported in the literature during the past 10 years (Tables 1a and b: sei-zure reduction per seizure type in corpus callosotomy and VNS; Table 2: seizure outcome in general after different approaches; Table 3: possible indications for pal-liative procedures depending on the leading seizure type or underlying syndrome). Moreover, some palliative procedures are suitable only for highly selected patient groups such as SEEG-guided thermocoagulation for patients undergoing invasive video-SEEG monitoring and MST for patients with an epileptogenic focus in elo-quent brain areas.

Third, the invasiveness of alternative palliative procedures varies considerably. The implantation of a VNS is a low-risk procedure compared to a corpus callosotomy. Anterior corpus callosotomy is less frequently associated with chronic disconnection syndromes than is complete corpus callosotomy; however, it is also less effective in reducing seizure severity and frequency. In patients with Lennox-Gastaut syndrome, for example, VNS and anterior or complete callosotomy are potentially alternative therapies. Identifying suitable candidates for each procedure remains challenging.

The decision is based on mainly individual criteria, a general consensus does not exist. Important individual features of the patients include the most disabling seizure type(s), the urge for immediate improvement (how many drop attacks? how many generalized tonic-clonic seizures?), presumed quality of life, intellectual performance, and the age of the patient. In some patients a two-step procedure is justified, beginning with a low-risk procedure and then, in case of failure, therapy with higher risks. It should be taken into consideration that it takes time for the maximal anticonvulsive effect of VNS to be seen. Procedures with a higher perioperative risk or risk of postoperative prolonged or permanent neurologic deficits are only legitimate if seizure outcome is supposed to be superior to less invasive procedures. This has been shown for complete corpus callosotomy versus anterior corpus callosotomy and is supposed for callosotomy versus VNS with respect to drop attacks and generalized tonic-clonic seizures.

The establishment of new therapeutic strategies such as deep/direct brain stimulation in medically intractable epilepsy is a most intriguing topic and will depend mainly on the proof of equality or superiority to well-known palliative procedures. Finally, cost-effectiveness (in particular that of individually tailored devices for responsive cortical stimulation) will not be just a marginal factor in the acceptance of these new therapeutic strategies.

Acknowledgements We thank Dr. Thomas Freiman, Department of Neurosurgery, University of Freiburg, Freiburg, Germany, for providing the Figures 1 to 4.

References

1. Aldenkamp AP, Majoie HJ, Berfelo MW, Evers SM, Kessels AG, Renier WO, Wilmink J (2002) Long-term effects of 24-month treatment with vagus nerve stimulation on behavior in children with Lennox-Gastaut syndrome. Epilepsy Behav 3:475–479
2. Alexopoulos AV, Kotagal P, Loddenkemper T, Hammel J, Bingaman WE (2006) Long-term results with vagus nerve stimulation in children with pharmacoresistant epilepsy. Seizure 15:491–503
3. Amar AP, Apuzzo ML, Liu CY (2004) Vagus nerve stimulation therapy after failed cranial surgery for intractable epilepsy: results from the vagus nerve stimulation therapy patient outcome registry. Neurosurgery 55:1086–1093
4. Amar AP, DeGiorgio CM, Tarver WB, Apuzzo ML (1999) Long-term multicenter experience with vagus nerve stimulation for intractable partial seizures: results of the XE5 trial. Stereotact Funct Neurosurg 73:104–108
5. Andrade DM, Zumsteg D, Hamani C, Hodaie M, Sarkissian S, Lozano AM, Wennberg RA (2006) Long-term follow-up of patients with thalamic deep brain stimulation for epilepsy. Neurology 66:1571–1573
6. Asadi-Pooya AA, Sharan A, Nei M, Sperling MR (2008) Corpus callosotomy. Epilepsy Behav 13:271–278
7. Bauman JA, Ridgway EB, Devinsky O, Doyle WK (2006) Subpectoral implantation of the vagus nerve stimulator. Neurosurgery 58(4 Suppl 2):ONS-322-5; discussion ONS-325-6
8. Benifla M, Otsubo H, Ochi A, Snead OC 3rd, Rutka JT (2006) Multiple subpial transection in pediatric epilepsy: indications and outcomes. Childs Nerv Syst 22:992–998
9. Benifla M, Rutka JT, Logan W, Donner EJ (2006) Vagal nerve stimulation for refractory epilepsy in children: indications and experience at the Hospital for Sick Children. Childs Nerv Syst 22:1018–1026

10. Ben-Menachem E, Hellstrom K, Waldton C, Augustinson LE (1999) Evaluation of refractory epilepsy treated with vagus nerve stimulation for up to 5 years. Neurology 52:1265–1267
11. Ben-Menachem E, Manon-Espaillat R, Ristanovic R, Wilder BJ, Stefan H, Mirza W, Tarver WB, Wernicke JF, for the First International Vagus Nerve Stimulation Study Group (1994) Vagus nerve stimulation for treatment of partial seizures: 1. A controlled study of effect on seizures. Epilepsia 35:616–626
12. Blount JP, Langburt W, Otsubo H, Chitoku S, Ochi A, Weiss S, Snead OC, Rutka JT (2004) Multiple subpial transections in the treatment of pediatric epilepsy. J Neurosurg 100:118–124
13. Boon P, Vonck K, De Herdt V, Van Dycke A, Goethals M, Goossens L, Van Zandijcke M, De Smedt T, Dewaele I, Achten R, Wadman W, Dewaele F, Caemaert J, Van Roost D (2007) Deep brain stimulation in patients with refractory temporal lobe epilepsy. Epilepsia 48:1551–1560
14. Buelow JM, Aydelott P, Pierz DM, Heck B (1996) Multiple subpial transection for Landau-Kleffner syndrome. AORN J 63:727–729, 732–735, 737–739, 741–744
15. Catenoix H, Mauguiere F, Guenot M, Ryvlin P, Bissery A, Sindou M, Isnard J (2008) SEEG-guided thermocoagulation: a palliative treatment of nonoperable partial epilepsies. Neurology 71(21):1719–1726
16. Celis MA, Moreno-Jiménez S, Lárraga-Gutiérrez JM, Alonso-Vanegas MA, García-Garduño OA, Martínez-Juárez IE, Fernández-Gónzalez MC (2007) Corpus callosotomy using conformal stereotactic radiosurgery. Childs Nerv Syst 23:917–920
17. Chabardes S, Kahane P, Minotti L, Koudsie A, Hirsch E, Benabid AL (2002) Deep brain stimulation in epilepsy with particular reference to the subthalamic nucleus. Epileptic Disord 4(Suppl 3):S83–S93
18. Charous SJ, Kempster G, Manders E, Ristanovic R (2001) The effect of vagal nerve stimulation on voice. Laryngoscope 111:2028–2031
19. Chervin RD, Pierce PA, Connors BW (1988) Periodicity and directionality in the propagation of epileptiform discharges across neocortex. J Neurophysiol 60:1695–1713
20. Chkhenkli SA, Sramaka M, Lortkipandize GS, Rakviashvili TN, Bregvadze ES, Magalashvili GE, Gagoshidze TS, Chkhenkeli IS (2004) Electrophysiological effects and clinical results of direct brain stimulation for intractable epilepsy. Clin Neurol Neurosurg 106:318–329
21. Cooper IS, Amin I, Gilman S (1973) The effect of chronic cerebellar stimulation upon epilepsy in man. Trans Am Neurol Assoc 98:192–196
22. Cross JH, Neville BG (2009) The surgical treatment of Landau-Kleffner syndrome. Epilepsia 50(Suppl 7):63–67
23. Cukiert A, Burattini JA, Mariani PP, Cukiert CM, Sárgentoni-Baldochi M, Baise-Zung C, Fortser CR, Mello VA (2009) Outcome after extended callosal section in patients with primary idiopathic generalized epilepsy. Epilepsia 50(6):1377–1380
24. Cukiert A, Burattini JA, Mariani PP, Câmara RB, Seda L, Baldauf CM, Argentoni M, Baise-Zung C, Forster CR, Mello VA (2006) Extended, one-stage callosal section for treatment of refractory secondarily generalized epilepsy in patients with Lennox-Gastaut and Lennox-like syndromes. Epilepsia 47:371–374
25. De Herdt V, Boon P, Ceulemans B, Hauman H, Lagae L, Legros B, Sadzot B, Van Bogaert P, van Rijckevorsel K, Verhelst H, Vonck K (2007) Vagus nerve stimulation for refractory epilepsy: a Belgian multicenter study. Eur J Paediatr Neurol 11:261–269
26. DeGiorgio C, Heck C, Bunch S, Britton J, Green P, Lancman M, Murphy J, Olejniczak P, Shih J, Arrambide S, Soss J (2005) Vagus nerve stimulation for epilepsy: randomized comparison of three stimulation paradigms. Neurology 65:317–319
27. DeGiorgio CM, Schachter SC, Handforth A, Salinsky M, Thompson J, Uthman B, Reed R, Collins S, Tecoma E, Morris GL, Vaughn B, Naritoku DK, Henry T, Labar D, Gilmartin R, Labiner D, Osorio I, Ristanovic R, Jones J, Murphy J, Ney G, Wheless J, Lewis P, Heck C (2000) Prospective long-term study of vagus nerve stimulation for the treatment of refratory seizures. Epilepsia 41:1195–1200
28. Eder HG, Feichtinger M, Pieper T, Kurschel S, Schroettener O (2006) Gamma knife radiosurgery for callosotomy in children with drug-resistant epilepsy. Childs Nerv Syst 22:1012–1017
29. Elliott RE, Morsi A, Kalhorn SP, Marcus J, Sellin J, Kang M, Silverberg A, Rivera E, Geller E, Carlson C, Devinsky O, Doyle WK (2011) Vagus nerve stimulation in 436 consecutive

patients with treatment-resistant epilepsy: long-term outcomes and predictors of response. Epilepsy Behav 20:57–63

30. Ergene E, Behr PK, Shih JJ (2001) Quality-of-life assessment in patients treated with vagus nerve stimulation. Epilepsy Behav 2:284–287

31. Feichtinger M, Schröttner O, Eder H, Holthausen H, Pieper T, Unger F, Holl A, Gruber L, Körner E, Trinka E, Fazekas F, Ott E (2006) Efficacy and safety of radiosurgical callosotomy: a retrospective analysis. Epilepsia 47:1184–1191

32. Fisher R, Salanova V, Witt T, Worth R, Henry T, Gross R, Oommen K, Osorio I, Nazzaro J, Labar D, Kaplitt M, Sperling M, Sandok E, Neal J, Handforth A, Stern J, DeSalles A, Chung S, Shetter A, Bergen D, Bakay R, Henderson J, French J, Baltuch G, Rosenfeld W, Youkilis A, Marks W, Garcia P, Barbaro N, Fountain N, Bazil C, Goodman R, McKhann G, Babu Krishnamurthy K, Papavassiliou S, Epstein C, Pollard J, Tonder L, Grebin J, Coffey R, Graves N, SANTE Study Group (2010) Electrical stimulation of the anterior nucleus of thalamus for treatment of refractory epilepsy. Epilepsia 51(5):899–908

33. Fisher RS, Uematsu S, Krauss G, Cysyk BJ, McPherson R, Lesser RP, Gordon B, Schwerdt P, Rise M (1992) Placebo-controlled pilot study of centromedian thalamic stimulation in treatment of intractable seizures. Epilepsia 33:841–851

34. Flanigin HF, Nashold BS (1976) Stereotactic lesions of the amygdala and hippocampus in epilepsy. Acta Neurochir 23:235–239

35. Fountas KN, Smith JR, Murro AM, Politsky J, Park YD, Jenkins PD (2005) Implantation of a closed-loop stimulation in the management of medically refractory focal epilepsy: a technical note. Stereotact Funct Neurosurg 83:153–158

36. Frost M, Gates J, Helmers SL, Wheless JW, Levisohn P, Tardo C, Conry JA (2001) Vagus nerve stimulation in children with refractory seizures associated with Lennox-Gastaut syndrome. Epilepsia 42:1148–1152

37. George R, for the Vagus Nerve Stimulation Study Group (1995) A randomized controlled trial of chronic vagus nerve stimulation for treatment of medically intractable seizures. Neurology 45:224–230

38. George R, Salinsky M, Kuzniecky R, Rosenfeld W, Bergen D, Tarver WB, Wernicke JF, for the First International Vagus Nerve Stimulation Study Group (1994) Vagus nerve stimulation for treatment of partial seizures: 3. Long-term follow-up on first 67 patients exiting a controlled study. Epilepsia 35:637–643

39. Grote CL, Van Slyke P, Hoeppner JA (1999) Language outcome following multiple subpial transections for Landau-Kleffner syndrome. Brain 122:561–566

40. Guenot M, Isnard J, Ryvlvlin P, Fischer C, Mauguiere F, Sindou M (2004) SEEG-guided RF thermocoagulation of epileptic foci: feasibility, safety, and preliminary results. Epilepsia 45:1368–1374

41. Haberler C, Alesch F, Mazal P, Pilz P, Jellinger K, Pinter MM, Hainfellner JA, Budka H (2000) No tissue damage by chronic deep brain stimulation in Parkinson's disease. Ann Neurol 48:372–376

42. Handforth A, DeGiorgio CM, Schachter SC, Uthman BM, Naritoku DK, Tecoma ES, Henry TR, Collins SD, Vaughn BV, Gilmartin RC, Labar DR, Morris GL 3rd, Salinsky MC, Osorio I, Ristanovic RK, Labiner DM, Jones JC, Murphy JV, Ney GC, Wheless JW (1998) Vagus nerve stimulation therapy for partial-onset seizures: a randomized active-control trial. Neurology 51:48–55

43. Hanson RR, Risinger M, Maxwell R (2002) The ictal EEG as a predictive factor for outcome following corpus callosum section in adults. Epilepsy Res 49:89–97

44. Harden CL, Pulver MC, Radvin LD, Nikolov B, Halper JP, Labar DR (2000) A pilot study of mood in epilepsy patients treated via vagus nerve stimulation. Epilepsy Behav 1:93–99

45. Helmers SL, Whenless JW, Frost M, Gates J, Levisohn P, Tardo C, Conry JA, Yalnizoglou D, Madsen JR (2001) Vagus nerve stimulation therapy in pediatric patients with refractory epilepsy: a retrospective study. J Child Neurol 16:843–848

46. Hodaie M, Wennberg RA, Dostrovsky JO, Lozano AM (2002) Chronic anterior thalamus stimulation for intractable epilepsy. Epilepsia 43:603–608

47. Hufnagel A, Zentner J, Fernandez G, Wolf HK, Schramm J, Elger CE (1997) Multiple subpial transection for control of epileptic seizures: effectiveness and safety. Epilepsia 38:678–688

48. Irwin K, Birch V, Lees J, Polkey C, Alarcon G, Binnie C, Smedley M, Baird G, Robinson RO (2001) Multiple subpial transections in Landau-Kleffner syndrome. Dev Med Child Neurol 43:248–252
49. Jalilian L, Limbrick DD, Steger-May K, Johnston J, Powers AK, Smyth MD (2010) Complete versus anterior two-third corpus callosotomy in children. Analysis of outcome. J Neurosurg Pediatr 6:257–266
50. Jea A, Vachhrajani S, Johnson KK, Rutka JT (2008) Corpus callosotomy in children with intractable epilepsy using frameless stereotactic neuronavigation: 12-year experience at the Hospital for Sick Children in Toronto. Neurosurg Focus 25:E7
51. Jea A, Vachhrajani S, Widjaja E, Nilsson D, Raybaud C, Shroff M, Rutka JT (2008) Corpus callosotomy in children and the disconnection syndromes: a review. Childs Nerv Syst 24:685–692
52. Jenssen S, Sperling MR, Tracy JI, Nei M, Joyce L, David G, O'Connor M (2006) Corpus callosotomy in refractory idiopathic generalized epilepsy. Seizure 15:621–629
53. Jobst BC, Darcey T, Bujarski KA, Thandani VM, Roberts DW (2009) Application of brief electrical pulses in the primary motor and supplementary motor cortex for the termination of after discharges. Epilepsia 50:2
54. Kerrigan JF, Litt B, Fisher RS, Cranstoun S, French JA, Blum DE, Dichter M, Shetter A, Baltuch G, Jaggi J, Krone S, Brodie M, Rise M, Graves N (2004) Electrical stimulation of the anterior nucleus of the thalamus for the treatment of intractable epilepsy. Epilepsia 45:346–354
55. Kim DS, Yang KH, Kim TG, Chang JH, Chang JW, Choi JU, Lee BI (2004) The surgical effect of callosotomy in the treatment of intractable seizures. Yonsei Med J 45:233–240
56. Kirse DJ, Werle AH, Murphy JV, Eyen TP, Bruegger DE, Hornig GW, Torkelson RD (2001) Vagus nerve stimulator implantation in children. Arch Otolaryngol Head Neck Surg 128:1263–1268
57. Kostov K, Kostov H, Tauboll E (2009) Long-term vagus nerve stimulation in the treatment of Lennox-Gastaut syndrome. Epilepsy Behav 16:321–324
58. Krahl SE, Clark KB, Smith DC, Browning RA (1998) Locus coeruleus lesions suppress the seizure-attenuating effect of vagus nerve stimulation. Epilepsia 39:709–714
59. Kwan P, Brodie MJ (2000) Early identification of refractory epilepsy. N Engl J Med 342:314–319
60. Kwan SY, Lin JH, Wong TT, Chang KP, Yiu CH (2006) A comparison of seizure outcome after callosotomy in patients with Lennox-Gastaut syndrome and positive or negative history of West syndrome. Seizure 15:552–557
61. Labar D (2004) Vagus nerve stimulation for 1 year in 269 patients on unchanged antiepileptic drugs. Seizure 13:392–398
62. Labar D, Murphy J, Tecoma E, for the E04 VNS Study Group (1999) Vagus nerve stimulation for medication-resistant generalized epilepsy. Neurology 52:1510–1512
63. Lega BC, Halpern CH, Jaggi JL, Baltuch GH (2010) Deep brain stimulation in the treatment of refractory epilepsy: update on the current data and future directions. Neurobiol Dis 38:354–360
64. Lesser RP, Kim SH, Beyderman L, Miglioretti DL, Webber WR, Bare M, Cysyk B, Krauss G, Gordon B (1999) Brief bursts of pulse stimulation terminate after discharges caused by cortical stimulation. Neurology 53:2073–2081
65. Liang S, Li A, Jiang H, Meng X, Zhao M, Zhang J, Sun Y (2010) Anterior corpus callosotomy in patients with intractable generalized epilepsy and mental retardation. Stereotact Funct Neurosurg 88:246–252
66. Lim SN, Lee ST, Tsai YT, Chen IA, Tu PH, Chen JL, Chang HW, Su YC, Wu T (2007) Electrical stimulation of the anterior nucleus of the thalamus for intractable epilepsy: a long-term follow-up study. Epilepsia 48:342–347
67. Loddenkemper T, Pan A, Neme S, Baker KB, Rezai AR, Dinner DS, Montgomery EB Jr, Lüders HO (2001) Deep brain stimulation in epilepsy. J Clin Neurophysiol 18:514–532

68. Lüders H, Schuele S (2006) Epilepsy surgery in patients with malformations of cortical development. Curr Opin Neurol 19:169–174
69. Lueders H, Bustamante LA, Zablow L, Goldensohn ES (1981) The independence of closely spaced discrete experimental spike foci. Neurology 31:846–851
70. Maehara T, Shimizu H (2001) Surgical outcome of corpus callosotomy in patients with drop attacks. Epilepsia 42:67–71
71. Maehara T, Shimizu H, Oda M, Arai N (1996) Surgical treatment of children with intractable epilepsy. Neurol Med Chir (Tokyo) 36:306–309
72. Majoie HJ, Berfelo MW, Aldenkamp AP, Evers SM, Kessels AG, Renier WO (2001) Vagus nerve stimulation in children with therapy-resistant epilepsy diagnosed as Lennox-Gastaut syndrome. J Clin Neurophysiol 18:419–428
73. Mamelak AN, Barbaro NM, Walker JA, Laxer KD (1993) Corpus callosotomy a quantitative study of extent of resection, seizure control, and neuropsychological outcome. J Neurosurg 79:688–695
74. Marino Junior R (1985) Surgery for epilepsy. Selective partial microsurgical callosotomy for intractable multiform seizures: criteria for clinical selection and results. Appl Neurophysiol 48:404–407
75. Marlow BA, Edwards J, Marzec M, Sagher O, Ross D, Fromes G (2001) Vagus nerve stimulation reduces daytime sleepiness in epilepsy patients. Neurology 57:879–884
76. Maxwell RE, Gates JR, Gumnit RJ (1986) Corpus callosotomy at the University of Minnesota. In: Engel J Jr (ed) Surgical treatment of epilepsies. Raven Press, New York, pp 659–666
77. McLachlan RS (1993) Suppression of interictal spikes and seizures by stimulation of the vagus nerve. Epilepsia 94:918–923
78. Mirski MA, Ferrendelli JA (1986) Anterior thalamic mediation of generalized pentylenetetrazol seizures. Brain Res 399:212–223
79. Mirski MA, Rossell LA, Terry JB, Fisher RS (1997) Anticonvulsant effect of anterior thalamic high frequency electrical stimulation in the rat. Epilepsy Res 28:89–100
80. Morrell F, Whisler WW, Smith MC, Hoeppner TJ, de Toledo-Morrell L, Pierre-Louis SJ, Kanner AM, Buelow JM, Ristanovic R, Bergen D et al (1995) Landau-Kleffner syndrome. Treatment with subpial intracortical transection. Brain 118:1529–1546
81. Morrell F, Whisler WW, Bleck TP (1989) Multiple subpial transection. A new approach to the surgical treatment of focal epilepsy. J Neurosurg 70:231–239
82. Morrell M, Hirsch L, Bergey G, Barkley G, Wharen R, Murro A, Fisch B, Rossi M, Labar D, Duckrow R, Sirven J, Drazkowski J, Worrell G, Gwinn R (2008) Long-term safety and efficacy of the RNS™ system in adults with medically intractable partial onset seizures. Epilepsia 49:480
83. Morris GL, Mueller MW (1999) Long-term treatment with vagus nerve stimulation in patients with refractory epilepsy. The vagus nerve stimulation study group E01-E05. Neurology 53:1731–1735
84. Mountcastel VB (1997) The columnar organization of the neocortex. Brain 120:701–722
85. Mountcastle VB (1957) Modality and topographic properties of single neurons of cat's somatic cortex. J Neurophysiol 20:408–434
86. Mulligan LP, Spencer DD, Spencer SS (2001) Multiple subpial transections: the Yale experience. Epilepsia 42:226–229
87. Murphy JV, for the Pediatric VNS Study Group (1999) Left vagal nerve stimulation in children with medically refractory epilepsy. J Pediatr 134:563–566
88. Murphy JV, Torkelson R, Dowler I, Simon S, Hudson S (2003) Vagal nerve stimulation in refractory epilepsy: the first 100 patients receiving vagal nerve stimulation at a pediatric center. Arch Pediatr Adolesc Med 157:260–264
89. Narabayashi H, Nago T, Saito Y, Yoshida M, Nagahata M (1963) Stereotaxic amygdalotomy for behavior disorders. Arch Neurol 9:1–16
90. Nei M, O'Connor M, Liporace J, Sperling MR (2006) Refractory generalized seizures: response to corpus callosotomy and vagal nerve stimulation. Epilepsia 47:115–122
91. Orbach D, Romanelli P, Devinsky O, Doyle W (2001) Late seizure recurrence after multiple subpial transections. Epilepsia 42:1316–1319

92. Osorio I, Overman J, Giftakis J, Wilkinson SB (2007) High frequency thalamic stimulation for inoperable mesial temporal epilepsy. Epilepsia 48:1561–1571

93. Parrent AG, Lozano AM (2000) Stereotactic surgery for temporal lobe epilepsy. Can J Neurol Sci. 27 Suppl 1:S79-84; discussion S92–6. Review.

94. Patwardhan RV, Strong B, Bebin EM, Mathisen J, Grabb PA (2000) Efficacy of vagal nerve stimulation in children with medically refractory epilepsy. Neurosurgery 47:1353–1357; discussion 1357–1358

95. Penry JK, Dean JC (1990) Prevention of intractable partial seizures by intermittent vagal stimulation in humans: preliminary results. Epilepsia 31(Suppl 2):S40–S43

96. Pinard JM, Delalande O, Chiron C, Soufflet C, Plouin P, Kim Y, Dulac O (1999) Callosotomy for epilepsy after West syndrome. Epilepsia 40:1727–1734

97. Polkey CE (2001) Multiple subpial transection: a clinical assessment. Int Rev Neurobiol 45:547–569

98. Purves SJ, Wada JA, Woodhurst WB (1995) Corpus callosum section for complex partial seizures. In: Reeves AG, Roberts DW (eds) Epilepsy and the corpus callosum 2. Advances in behavioral biology, vol 45. Plenum, New York, pp 175–182

99. Purves SJ, Wada JA, Woodhurst WB, Moyes PD, Strauss E, Kosaka B, Li D (1988) Results of anterior corpus callosum section in 24 patients with medically intractable seizures. Neurology 38:1194–1201

100. Rahimi SY, Park YD, Witcher MR, Lee KH, Marrufo M, Lee MR (2007) Corpus callosotomy for treatment of pediatric epilepsy in the modern era. Pediatr Neurosurg 43:202–208

101. Rathore C, Abraham M, Rao RM, George A, Sankara Sarma P, Radhakrishnan K (2007) Outcome after corpus callosotomy in children with injurious drop attacks and severe mental retardation. Brain Dev 29:577–585

102. Reeves AG, Risse G (1995) Neurological effects of callosotomy. In: Reeves AG, Roberts DW (eds) Epilepsy and the corpus callosum 2. Advances in behavioral biology, vol 45. Plenum, New York, pp 241–251

103. Reichenthal E, Hocherman S (1977) The critical cortical area for development of penicillin-induced epilepsy. Electroencephalogr Clin Neurophysiol 42:248–251

104. Renfroe JB, Wheless JW (2002) Earlier use of adjunctive nerve stimulation therapy for refractory epilepsy. Neurology 59:S26–S30

105. Rosenfeld WE, Roberts DW (2009) Tonic and atonic seizures: what's next – VNS or callosotomy? Epilepsia 50(suppl 8):25–30

106. Rougier A, Sundstorm L, Claverie B, Saint-Hilaire JM, Labrecque R, Lurton D, Bouvier G (1996) Multiple subpial transection: report of 7 cases. Epilepsy Res 24:57–63

107. Rutecki P (1990) Anatomical, physiological, and theoretical basis for the antiepileptic effect of vagus nerve stimulation. Epilepsia 31(suppl 2):S1–S6

108. Sawhney IM, Robertson IJ, Polkey CE, Binnie CD, Elwes RD (1995) Multiple subpial transection: a review of 21 cases. J Neurol Neurosurg Psychiatry 58:344–349

109. Schachter SC (2002) Vagus nerve stimulation therapy summary: five years after FDA approval. Neurology 59(6 Suppl 4):S15–20. Review

110. Scherrmann J, Hoppe C, Kral T, Schramm J, Elger CE (2001) Vagus nerve stimulation: clinical experience in a large patient series. J Clin Neurophysiol 18:408–414

111. Schramm J, Aliashkevich AF, Grunwald T (2002) Multiple subpial transections: outcome and complications in 20 patients who did not undergo resection. J Neurosurg 97:39–47

112. Shahwan A, Bailey C, Maxiner W, Harvey AS (2009) Vagus nerve stimulation for refractory epilepsy in children: more to VNS than seizure frequency reduction. Epilepsia 50:1220–1228

113. Shimizu H (2005) Our experience with pediatric epilepsy surgery focusing on corpus callosotomy and hemispherectomy. Epilepsia 46(suppl 1):30–31

114. Shimizu H, Maehara T (2000) Neuronal disconnection for the surgical treatment of pediatric epilepsy. Epilepsia 41(Suppl 9):28–30

115. Smyth MD, Klein EE, Dodson WE, Mansur DB (2007) Radiosurgical posterior corpus callosotomy in a child with Lennox-Gastaut syndrome. J Neurosurg 106(4 Suppl):312–315

116. Smyth MD, Tubbs RS, Bebin EM, Grabb PA, Blount JP (2003) Complications of chronic of chronic vagus nerve stimulation for epilepsy in children. J Neurosurg 99:500–503
117. Spencer SS, Schramm J, Wyler A, O'Connor M, Orbach D, Krauss G, Sperling M, Devinsky O, Elger C, Lesser R, Mulligan L, Westerveld M (2002) Multiple subpial transection for intractable partial epilepsy: an international meta-analysis. Epilepsia 43:141–145
118. Sunaga S, Shimizu H, Sugano H (2009) Long-term follow-up of seizure outcomes after corpus callosotomy. Seizure 18:124–128
119. Tanriverdi T, Olivier A, Poulin N, Andermann F, Dubeau F (2009) Long-term seizure outcome after corpus callosotomy: a retrospective analysis of 95 patients. J Neurosurg 110:332–342
120. Tatum WOT, Helmers SL (2009) Vagus nerve stimulation and magnet use: optimizing benefits. Epilepsy Behav 15:299–302
121. Tellez-Zenteno JF, Dhar R, Wiebe S (2005) Long-term seizure outcomes following epilepsy surgery: a systematic review and meta-analysis. Brain 128:1188–1198
122. Tellez-Zenteno JF, McLachlan RS, Parrent A, Kubu CS, Wiebe S (2006) Hippocampal electrical stimulation in mesial temporal lobe epilepsy. Neurology 66:1490–1494
123. Turanli G, Yalnizoglu D, Genc-Acikgoz D, Akalan N, Topcu M (2006) Outcome and long-term follow-up after corpus callosotomy in childhood onset intractable epilepsy. Childs Nerv Syst 22:1322–1327
124. Uthman BM, Reichl AM, Dean JC, Eisenschenk S, Gilmore R, Reid S, Roper SN, Wilder BJ (2004) Effectiveness of vagus nerve stimulation in epilepsy patients: a 12-year observation. Neurology 63:1124–1126
125. Van Buren JM, Wood JH, Oakley J, Hambrecht F (1978) Preliminary evaluation of cerebellar stimulation by double-blind stimulation and biological criteria in the treatment of epilepsy. J Neurosurg 48:407–416
126. Van Wagenen WP, Herren RY (1940) Surgical division of commisural pathways in the corpus callosum: relation to spread of an epileptic attack. Arch Neurol Psychiatry 44:740–759
127. Velasco AL, Velasco F, Jimenez F, Velasco M, Castro G, Carrillo-Ruiz JD, Fanghänel G, Boleaga B (2006) Neuromodulation of the centromedian thalamic nuclei in the treatment of generalized seizures and the improvement of qualitiy of life in patients with Lennox-Gastaut syndrome. Epilepsia 47:1203–1212
128. Velasco AL, Velasco M, Velasco F, Trejo D, Castro G, Carrillo-Ruiz JD (2007) Electrical stimulation of the hippocampal epileptic foci for seizure control: a double-blind, long-term follow-up study. Epilepsia 48:1895–1903
129. Velasco F, Carrillo-Ruiz JD, Brito F, Velasco M, Velasco AL, Marquez I, Davis R (2005) Double-blind, randomized controlled pilot study of bilateral cerebellar stimulation for treatment of intractable motor seizures. Epilepsia 46:1071–1081
130. Velasco F, Velasco M, Ogarrio C, Fanghanel G (1987) Electrical stimulation of the centromedian thalamic nucleus in the treatment of convulsive seizures: a preliminary report. Epilepsia 28:421–430
131. Vonck K, Thadani V, Gilbert K, Dedeurwaerdere S, De Groote L, De Herdt V, Goossens L, Gossiaux F, Achten E, Thiery E, Vingerhoets G, Van Roost D, Caemaert J, De Reuck J, Roberts D, Williamson P, Boon P (2004) Vagus nerve stimulation for refractory epilepsy: a transatlantic experience. J Clin Neurophysiol 21:283–289
132. Vonck K, Van LK, Dedeurwaerdere S, Caemaert J, De RJ, Boon P (2001) The mechanism of action of vagus nerve stimulation for refractory epilepsy: the current status. J Clin Neurophysiol 18:394–401
133. Wadman WJ, Gutnick MJ (1993) Non-uniform propagation of epileptiform discharge in brain slices of rat neocortex. Neuroscience 52:255–262
134. Wheless JW (2009) Managing severe epilepsy syndromes of early childhood. J Child Neurol 24:24S–32S
135. Wille C, Steinhoff BJ, Altenmüller DM, Staak AM, Bilic SB, Nikkhah G, Vesper J (2011) Chronic high-frequency deep-brain stimulation in progressive myoclonic epilepsy in adulthood – report of five cases. Epilepsia 52(3):489–496

136. Wilson DH, Culver C, Waddington M, Gazzaniga M (1975) Disconnection of the cerebral hemispheres. An alternative to hemispherectomy for the control of intractable seizures. Neurology 25:1149–1153
137. Wilson DH, Reeves A, Gazzaniga M, Culver C (1977) Cerebral commissurotomy for control of intractable seizures. Neurology 27:708–715
138. Wong TT, Kwan SY, Chang KP, Hsiu-Mei W, Yang TF, Chen YS, Yi-Yen L (2006) Corpus callosotomy in children. Childs Nerv Syst 22:999–1011
139. Wright GD, McLellan DL, Brice JG (1994) A double-blind trial of chronic cerebellar stimulation in twelve patients with severe epilepsy. J Neurol Neurosurg Psychiatry 47:769–774
140. Zachnetti A, Wang SC, Moruzzi G (1952) The effect of vagal afferent stimulation on the EEG pattern of the cat. Electroencephalogr Clin Neurophysiol 4:357–361
141. Zentner J (1997) Surgical aspects of corpus callosum section. In: Tuxhorn I, Holthausen H, Boenigk H (eds) Paediatric epilepsy syndromes and their surgical treatment. John Libbey, London, pp 830–849

Author Index Volume 1–39

N. Akalan, C. Di Rocco (eds.), *Pediatric Epilepsy Surgery*,
Advances and Technical Standards in Neurosurgery,
DOI 10.1007/978-3-7091-1360-8, © Springer-Verlag Wien 2012

Subject Index Volume 1–39

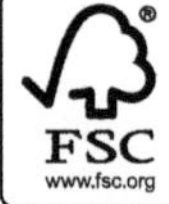

MIX
Papier aus verantwortungsvollen Quellen
Paper from responsible sources
FSC® C105338

If you have any concerns about our products,
you can contact us on
ProductSafety@springernature.com

In case Publisher is established outside the EU,
the EU authorized representative is:
Springer Nature Customer Service Center GmbH
Europaplatz 3, 69115 Heidelberg, Germany

Printed by Libri Plureos GmbH
in Hamburg, Germany